Aspects of
Homeopathy

Musculo-Skeletal
Problems

Ian Watson

Further copies of this book and other titles may be ordered at
www.cuttingedgepublications.co.uk

All enquiries should be addressed to
mail@cuttingedgepublications.co.uk

First printed in 1998. This edition published in 2004 by
Cutting Edge Publications
PO Box 32
Kendal
Cumbria
LA9 4AR

A catalogue record for this book is
available from the British Library

ISBN 0 9517657 4 4

Musculo-Skeletal Problems

A seminar with

Ian Watson

Dedication

This book is dedicated to Satpreet Grewal,
whose shining spirit touched all those
who were present at this seminar.

Preface

This is more or less a verbatim transcript of a one-day seminar that took place in San Anselmo, California in 1997. The actual transcribing was done by Carol Nelson, to whom I am especially grateful. I know for sure that left to my own devices I would never have gotten around to it. I have polished the text just enough to render it readable, without significantly altering the original content in any way. The style, as you will discover, remains colloquial and somewhat free-flowing. On reading it through, I was struck by the high level of interaction and discussion that took place during the day, and all of the questions and comments that were picked up by the tape recorder have been included here. Superfluous ramblings, repetitions and potentially libellous slips of the tongue have been carefully edited out. If you enjoy those parts, you will have to buy the tapes!

I have added a therapeutic index at the back of the book to help the reader locate specific musculo-skeletal problems, and a few other things besides. I've also added some subject headings here and there. I trust the reader will understand that this is not meant to be a comprehensive therapeutics book. It is simply a written record of what emerged on a particular day with a lively and unique audience. I am conscious that many more remedies and conditions could be added, but to do so would destroy the uniqueness of this particular work. It is, I feel, complete in itself.

The first version of this book was printed experimentally in 1998 without an ISBN number, as I was unconvinced there would be much demand for it. Happily, I have been proved wrong and the initial print run was entirely sold out, with demand increasing as time went on. Consequently, I have decided to re-publish it with an ISBN listing alongside my other titles.

Ian Watson
Summer 2004

Introduction

It's such a lovely day......I know you'd all rather be sunbathing or hanging out on the grass, but we're here to study, do a bit of work, and hopefully have a bit of fun, too. So those of you who don't know me, I'm Ian Watson. I'm a homeopath, kind of, from England. I say kind of, because I've been travelling so much the last couple of years, I haven't been in one place long enough to run a practice for a while, but I did practice for about eight years, non-stop. I trained in London, in England, and I was lucky to study with some really good classical homeopaths, but also with some really good eclectic practitioners as well. One of the things I've noticed is that you can do a lot with homeopathy that's outside of the range of the straight, classical, constitutional stuff, and so I've always kept that in mind in my own practice.

One of the things I've found in terms of building up a practice, especially in the beginning, is that there's plenty of room for specialization in homeopathy, and I think homeopaths generally are a bit against specialisation. We all try to be everything to all people, and there's nothing wrong with getting good in a particular area and sharing your expertise in that. So, with that in mind, I chose two specific topics for this weekend, to do some depth in a particular area. I mean, we could do a whole week on musculo-skeletal complaints, no problem. As it is, we've got a day.

What I hope for those of you not that familiar with this way of working is that you'll at least be able to have quite a lot of stuff at your fingertips, because the thing, particularly with trauma, when you're treating trauma to the body, is that you need to be able to respond to what's happening right there in front of you. Often, by the time you've gone home and switched the computer on and got the repertory out, it's too late. You missed it. They're down to the emergency ward already or they're having surgery or they're having something else. So there's a case to be made I think for getting some basic knowledge realy well assimilated, getting so familiar with it that it's literally at your fingertips. You see a situation and the remedy just comes to you. You think: *"where did that come from?"* and then you become like a compulsive prescriber, and people you don't even know, you find yourself giving them remedies. And you see all kinds of amazing things happen.

So what we'll do today, some of it I'm sure will be remedies you already know. I thought long and hard during the week prior to the seminar as to whether I could leave out some of the basics, the *Arnica* and the *Rhus-tox.*, and so on. Now, I don't intend to bore you with things you already know, but I do want to remind you of the importance of some of those things, because I think sometimes when we get into classical homeopathy and constitutional homeopathy, we think that's more important, and I don't think it is. I remember Robin Murphy saying that he thought the highest level of homeopathy, in his opinion, was first-aid, and the more I thought about it, the more I agreed with him. It's the most immediate. It's also the easiest, the most demonstrable, you need the least amount of training and skill, so it's the most teachable to other people.

It's in all of our interest that more people get homeopathy, at whatever level they get it. It's in all our interest that people just get a sense that homeopathy works, and what pulls most people into homeopathy is what I call an *Arnica* experience. You know, where they have no knowledge of homeopathy, don't know the first thing about it, but somebody catches them when they're susceptible. They've sprained their ankle, or they've got a bruise or a bang on the head, or something like that. Someone catches them in that moment and gives them a dose of *Arnica*, and they feel the effects. That person can never go back to being an allopath fully. It's like they'll never be well since that experience!

A lot of people don't get that from constitutional treatment. You know they go and maybe have a lengthy case-taking and get asked what seems to them a lot of irrelevant questions and pay a lot of money in some situations, and wait a long time for this one pill that didn't seem to do much. A lot of people have that as their first experience, then they can often conclude that homeopathy didn't work. And that's really sad. And yet a beginner could have given them *Arnica* in a first-aid situation, and they would have had a dramatic experience. I want to remind you that the emphasis is sometimes a bit unbalanced. We put too much importance on the constitutional approach.

Aetiologies

The other reason why I think Robin is right is that so many chronic health problems stem back to what were essentially first-aid situations. You know, "three years ago, I had a whiplash, I had a bang on the head, I sprained my ankle, I had a grief, I had a shock, a child fell off a swing," or something of this kind, and they've never been well since. You see a train of health problems. So I'm going to emphasise to you the importance of knowing the aetiologies of remedies, the causations, and knowing what the main remedies are for each aetiological situation. If you can think in terms of aetiologies, you don't have to remember symptoms nearly so much. This, you'll learn throughout the day, is the focus of my approach to musculo-skeletal therapeutic work. It's to concentrate on aetiological prescribing, i.e., finding out what was it that put the person into that state. Something impacted on their life and they've never been well since.

So the aetiologies are very important, in other words, what happened. Let's talk about that a little bit first of all. It's very important that if someone's in an accident that involved a bruising or a physical injury of some kind, I never assume that therefore that person will need *Arnica* two years later. And if they say that their health problems date back to that accident, what I want to know is, what did they take from that accident? To me, it's like they went into a take-away. Do you have take-away's here? What do you call it here?

Audience: Carry-out!

Ian: Carry-out. So you go into a carry-out - that's the trauma, that's what happened, but what did they carry out with them? What did they get to go, to take away? That's the question you really want to know. It's the combination of those two things that give us an aetiological prescription. What happened is the first thing you want to know, and the next thing is what did they take away?

And even more important than that, has what they took away had a lasting impact on their health? Because we have to also remember that people heal many things on their own. The vital force is intelligent and self-healing. I don't have the approach that you look at someone's history, and everybody who has had a bang on the head in their whole life, everybody therefore needs *Arnica*. There's a school of homeopathy that works that way, which I don't agree with. But if there's been a genuine trauma and it had an impact which was lasting, if the answer is yes, then that person needs an aetiological prescription, first and foremost. Which means that the remedy has to match the causation first, and only the symptoms, second. And if we don't get it that way around, then what tends to happen is palliation rather than cure, even with what would otherwise be considered good prescribing.

I've often seen it appear a bit like this - can you imagine the person's general picture is this - they're putting out mostly general symptoms: mentals, emotionals, physical generals, food desires, the things that we routinely take in a case history. But somewhere in that person's history, say they broke their leg, or they got concussed, or they had a big grief, or something of that kind. Very often there will be a mini-picture that they've carried with them ever since that time, and what I've found is that the well-indicated constitutional remedy will often fail until they've had this remedy. And that can be very puzzling if you're searching for that elusive one remedy that's going to cure everything and change the person's life.

It may be that you've found it, but the person can't benefit from it yet because they still have the sprained ankle or they still have neck problems since a whiplash. And those of you who are body-workers will know this, sometimes people can't heal, for example, on an emotional level until they have the body fixed. And it works both ways. So aetiology is very important. I want to run through with you some of the main aetiologies affecting the musculo-skeletal system, and for those of you who use the repertory, some places where you can find them. We'll talk about that a bit.

Affinities

The second thing I want to emphasise today is the importance of affinities. In other words, which organs and tissues are specifically affected by which remedies. I've found this to be one of the simplest ways to access the materia medica without having to learn a huge volume of information. So for me, knowing an affinity is worth knowing ten symptoms, approximately. I mean, that's a generalisation, but the principle is true. If you know one good affinity, I would rather know that than know ten symptoms of the same remedy. And I find it will help me more often. The fact that I know that *Ruta* has a primary affinity with the tendons, for example, is more useful to me than the fact that the person may have pain worse sitting, pain worse standing, pain worse walking, pain worse damp. You can have a list of symptoms which can still only get you down to three, four or five remedies, but the affinity can get you down to one remedy, or one or two, without any symptoms, so that's worth knowing to me. It's a question of efficiency.

The most efficient homeopath that I ever came across in the literature was Boger. All of you heard of Boger? Most of you? He's one of your own. He was American, I think, a homeopath, a great prescriber, and his skill was to select the highest quality, least quantity information, so he could home in on that small amount of information that, if you

4

prescribed on that, you would make accurate prescriptions. And the basis of his work was affinities. If you read his book, *Boger's Synoptic Key*, he was the first one to systematically list the organ and tissue affinities, and to give the kind of strength, the relative strength of each affinity, under every remedy. So for *Arnica*, he would say soft tissues first, then muscles, then bones, then blood, and so on. He'd actually grade them. He'd say, this is the most important, and it's also got these ones.

He must have trained himself to think that way, and when you have the ability to do that, when you look at a case, you can see where this particular pathology is coming from. Where is the disturbance right now? Ahh, it's soft tissues, it's cellular tissues, it's the serous membranes, it's the muscle, it's the bone. In the process of doing that, a bunch of remedies should come to mind, and you know that you're in the right group already. And with a bit of practice, you can do that even while you're taking a case, even on the telephone, without opening any books or anything. As the patient is speaking, you think, "O.K., I'm into this group. I know what group I'm in." The beauty of working this way is that whilst still taking the case now, having got down to a relevant group, you can ask leading questions to differentiate which remedy is needed. So you think it's between *Calc.-phos.*, *Symphytum*, *Calc.-carb.* and *Ruta*. So now you can ask some *Ruta* questions, you can ask some *Calc.-phos.* questions, and you can eliminate the remedies that don't fit quite quickly.

All of the best homeopaths I've studied with asked loads of leading questions during their case taking. And I was taught at college that you're not supposed to do that - and you were too, right? And yet when I went and sat in with people who were actually really good, who didn't just teach it but were actually seeing 20-30 people a day and being really effective and being appropriate prescribers, in other words, they were treating people on the level that they wanted treating, which isn't always what the homeopath thought wanted treating, when I worked with people who were doing that, what I saw they had in common was that they could ask direct leading questions during the interview, and so they could differentiate remedies before the case-taking was over. What that meant was, nine times out of ten, they didn't have to take the case home and work on it. They did the work there and then, during the visit. It's very practical, and it's very cost-effective in terms of the practitioner's time and energy. You should be able to do the job when you're on the job. I don't think it's that efficient that homeopaths routinely take all their cases home and do another day in the clinic at home, which you're not being paid for. It's not good marketing, is it, Satpreet? We should do it while we're in the clinic, I think.

Case Analysis

Those are the things I emphasise. Having said that, occasionally it's that strange, rare and peculiar symptom that helps you more than anything. So I'm not saying: "throw out the symptomatic approach." What I am saying is: "put it in its right place." Symptoms, in my opinion, should be secondary to aetiologies and affinities. They shouldn't be the most important thing. If you start your case analysis by looking at a list of symptoms, there's something missing. There's a step that you missed out. What it means is that you didn't understand what you were treating. If you just take a list of symptoms and start matching those symptoms to rubrics, what that means is you haven't got clear on what you're treating yet. You're just doing symptom-matching, and that's like, how can you say it without being offensive? That's like kindergarten homeopathy. It's not really perceiving what has to be cured, which Hahnemann emphasised over and over and over again. Perceiving what has to be cured means you understand what you're treating before you start doing any real analysis. Once you've got that understanding, the analysis is automatic. You know what you're working on.

Any questions on that bit? It's fairly straightforward.

Jane: Seems like it would make sense to apply that to constitutional treatment, too?
Ian: Yes, I think in any case, affinities are highly valuable, in absolutely any case, and I find it helps me whatever level I'm treating on, whether it be miasmatic, constitutional, organ affinity, and I include under affinities that it may be that it's an emotional affinity. You know, if you take the case, and what you perceive is that the person's energy is tied up more in an emotional state, even though they've got physical problems, then you know that you need a remedy that has emotional issues first, physical things second. The same principle still applies.

We've got a case example that illustrates that. In fact, I can think of a few that illustrate that. Some people will come in, you body workers will know, people will come in and they'll say that they've got a back problem, right? And you work on their back for six months, and they still seem to have it. Or every time you fix it, it goes again.

Any of you in body work will know that people have this pattern sometimes. And sooner or later, you perceive that there's something underlying. There's a predisposition for their back to keep going, or for whatever it is that keeps happening, for that muscle to go into spasm or something. And it may be that what they really need is an emotional-based prescription. In which case, working on their back is like level one, but it won't get them cured. What you need is to go underneath that, and the sooner that you can do that, the better for the patient. But sometimes it takes a while, and I think we have to work our way in and you have to build up trust with the person, and so on and so forth. And most people come in with one problem, and it's not always the real reason why they came. But yes, I think you're right, Jane, the principle applies on any level of prescribing.

So what I'll do with you today, I want to do a combination of remedies that you're familiar with in the first aid sense, in the traumatic sense, and remedies which are more constitutional, which have a tendency to certain musculoskeletal problems. I want to talk about some that I've had a lot of experience with. And also, I want to talk about some little remedies which you can add to the ones that you already know, if you're not familiar with them. There's a whole range of remedies that have just got very specific therapeutic actions, remedies like *Thiosiaminum*, for example. You couldn't run a practice without *Thiosiaminum*, could you? (Laughter.) So ones like that I want to talk about. They're tiny, a little paragraph in Boericke somewhere, and yet, if you know what they do well, they are so useful. So there are little ones like that which I want to throw in. Now everybody's looking up *Thiosiaminum* (laughter).

Bone Remedies

So I want to talk about some bone issues with you first of all. That's the first affinity that we're going to have a look at. There's a few categories of things that I want to look at with bones, and if any of you have any questions or things you've seen in practice and you've maybe struggled to treat it or you wonder about treating it, feel free to ask me, and I'll try and respond. I'll talk to you about fractures of different kinds, injuries to bones. I also want to talk about bone pains, and we'll also touch on bone cancer, tumours and growths, exostoses, spurs, that kind of thing.

7

Fractures

So we've got some fracture remedies here, and one of the things that I learned after a while, treating first-aid, is that the normal rules that apply to constitutional prescribing, don't apply to first-aid prescribing, like to give one dose of the 30c and then see the patient a month later and see how they're doing. It's out the window. It's completely inappropriate.

From my own experience, I learned quite quickly that if you want to demonstrate that homeopathy can be really effective in first aid, you have to be - I don't want to use the word aggressive - but you have to be pretty on the ball when you're prescribing, and you have to be very prepared to repeat frequently, to give high potencies frequently, if it's needed, and to change the remedy frequently. If you're doing single remedy homeopathy, you need to be willing to switch from one remedy to another, as each remedy deals with its aspect of that trauma. If someone has a fracture, then you have bone damage, obviously. You also have soft tissue damage. You have probably got muscular inflammation and pain and there's going to be bleeding, some internal haemorrhage. There may be an open sore or wound that needs taking care of. That could be five different remedies, all in the space of forty-eight hours, you may need to take the person through those. So, those of you who are not familiar with treating in that way, I just want to give you permission to do that, and remind you that it's actually necessary. It's appropriate.

We generally, routinely, need to start with *Arnica*, and the reason being, as much as anything, it's not because *Arnica* has a primary affinity with the bone, but because *Arnica* has a primary affinity with shock, with people who are in shock. And anybody who's had a fracture or an injury of that kind is going to be in shock. The body is going to be in shock, even if the person isn't.

Here's one little tip with *Arnica*, that I've seen with children in particular. I can remember vividly a case of a boy I've treated, I just happened to be there, when a boy came back, he'd been playing, he was screaming. He had fallen out of a tree, or something like that, and had landed on his arm. His arm was obviously in a great deal of pain. He was holding it like this. I was at the person's house and the Mom had a first aid kit in the house, and we both looked at him, and we said, *"Arnica,"* straight away. We started dosing the boy with *Arnica* 200's every few minutes, and pretty quickly, he calmed down and felt the arm, and it felt fine. And he was like, *"I'll see you at tea time, Mom."* He wanted to be off.

We both had this feeling of, *"hang on a minute - that looked pretty serious."* The response to the *Arnica* was so rapid and so quick that he seemed O.K. He'd actually fractured his arm. It was not a particularly bad fracture, but he'd got a fracture in his arm, which surely would have showed up in a few days. Had we taken his word for it, he'd have been off running again, and he would have been in trouble a couple of days down the line.

So it's important to remember that remedies can be so effective that they can sometimes mask an underlying problem. They give such quick and rapid pain relief that this is why perceiving what has to be cured is really important. Once we examined him, the fact that his arm actually bent both ways with virtually no pain - that was the amazing thing. He's like, *"Oh yeah, isn't that strange!"* which demonstrated that he had a problem there. He actually needed a cast and so on, so one of the important things is getting to the hospital and getting the arm set.

The thing with treating fractures is that it's really important to get the arm set before we start giving remedies that speed up the healing. I know that you all know this, but I've done it. I've done it the other way and I know people who've done it the other way. They read in the book, *"Symphytum* to set fractures," and before they've even got the bone set properly, they're dosing the kid with *Symphytum*, so that bone is now set and it's out here somewhere. I know two people from my own practice where they've had to go back and have it rebroken and reset, which is not nice. It's worth avoiding having that done.

Audience: With the *Arnica* 200, you said that you gave it every few minutes - really?

Ian: Yes. Absolutely.

Audience: Every five or ten minutes until he stopped screaming?

Ian: Yes.

Audience: Or even higher or more frequent? Would you have given higher than that?

Ian: Two hundred was what they had in the house. If it had been 1M or 10M, it would have been the same for me.

I'll tell you how I learned that. It was from my own experience. Before I got into homeopathy, I had a bad ankle sprain, and I knew nothing about remedies, and it took me probably about a year to heal it. When I first got into homeopathy, I sprained my ankle ;again, and all I knew then was 6's and 30's, so I took *Arnica* 6 three times a day, which is what it said on the bottle for this ankle sprain, which was pretty bad. It made no impact whatsoever, and my conclusion was that *Arnica* didn't work. It took me eighteen months to heal that one.

When I'd practised homeopathy for a while, I did the same thing again, same ankle, really bad sprain. It was probably the worst one. By this time, I had experience treating other people. So my ankle is out here somewhere, really badly swollen. It was probably six hours before I could get to a place where I could start treating it. I was away from home, or whatever, and so I started taking *Arnica* 10M's. I took it first of all every five minutes, every ten minutes, every fifteen, every half hour, until I felt that it was starting to really work. It wasn't until I'd had maybe five or six doses that I even felt it do something. And within twenty-four hours, there was no sign that I'd ever sprained it. So what was previously eighteen months, or twelve months, the whole thing was healed in twenty-four hours, just on that *Arnica*. And also I was using it externally. By this time I knew about external things as well, so I was using *Arnica* ointment externally, and so on. It's quite hard to overdose in first aid situations. This has been my experience. It's very hard, and I would include burns. Err on the side of over-prescribing, initially, until you see there's a really good response, and then you can back off. Sometimes you really need to push it. Similarly with high fevers and stuff like that. Anything where there's a lot of intensity going on, a very acute high fever. You've got a child with a 102, 103 fever. They'll burn the remedy up so fast, you'll think you gave them the wrong remedy. You start chopping and changing, and what they actually needed was more of it. More of it, higher potency, more of it. It's not always the case, but if you don't see a response to your first remedy, give it again, give it again, at least in first-aid situations. I've had much better results doing that.

Treating Acutes

Audience: This is a little off the subject but what would you think about a case where a young child has a very high fever and it looks like a very clear case of *Belladonna* and the child gets one dose of 12c, and the whole thing is gone?

Ian: Yes, you'll see that too. I've talked about this before. There's no contradiction there. Every acute is self-limiting, by definition. An acute disease has a cycle. There's a beginning, a middle and an end, and depending on when you start the treatment, that will also help to determine the response of the child. So if you see that result, one dose of 12c and everything's blown away, the chances are this is the point at which you gave it.

Audience: Toward the beginning?

Ian: There are two places where you can abort something quickly: one is, if this is the start point, and you give the remedy right here, then you can abort the whole thing. It's as if it never happened. You just blow it away with the first dose. But, if the disease has already progressed, then there's a point of no return which is reached. If you prescribe anywhere beyond here, it will get worse before it gets better, probably. They'll need to go through it. You'll see this with the measles and the mumps and the childhood acutes and all these things. There's a certain point at which, even though you gave them the right remedy, all you can do is shorten the time now. You can't abort it. They've got to complete it. You'll see they'll go through it in what would have been four days, they'll do it in maybe two days, or twenty-four hours, or something like that. If you prescribe towards the end of the cycle, you'll see very rapid cure on one dose again, because they were nearly there anyway. So if you prescribe close to the beginning or close to the end, it's like you'll blow it away. But there's a cut-off point either side of that. That's the way I visualise it.

That's why people don't always respond the same way in acutes. It has nothing to do with giving the right remedy, the wrong remedy, or even the right potency or wrong potency. It's more to do with where they were at in the disease cycle when you began the treatment. So, in the case that you just mentioned, where would they be?

Audience: I think that she was pretty close to the beginning. They usually call me up pretty quick.

Ian: Yes. You catch something right at the onset, this is like the first sneeze, you give that *Aconite*, and boom, it's gone. The next morning they're fine. If you wait until they're already coughing and it's gone down to their chest, *Aconite* won't even work. They'll have to go through *Hepar* or *Spongia* or something like that. So there's something to be said for having the remedies in the house, right? That's what you learn about first-aid and acute prescribing. There's no substitute for having the remedies there and then, and they take it on the spot, preferably before they even call you. I mean, I would endeavour to train your patient to at least give the remedy they think before they even call you. If someone rings up and they say, "It's right-sided and it's hot and it's throbbing and it started at 3:00 o'clock", if they haven't given *Belladonna*, I'd want to know why not! They should be able to do that. Patients shouldn't need to be dependent on homeopaths for that level of prescribing.

Audience: I've got them to that place with *Arnica*.
Ian: That's a good place to start.

Fractures Continued......

Let's just quickly talk about a few of these other remedies. *Bryonia*, I learned, is one of the best pain-relieving remedies when there's been a fracture situation. So this is often a better pain reliever than *Arnica*. *Arnica* may well take care of the bruising and stop the bleeding and bring them out of shock, but if a person's in a great deal of pain and sensitivity, *Bryonia*, and the other one that's not on this list but you can add it, is *Hepar*, may be needed. You really only need the modality to differentiate. So if you've got worse from the slightest movement as a modality, then give *Bryonia*. And again, high potencies repeated if someone's broken a leg or fractured a hip or something of this kind. They're on the way to the hospital, *Bryonia* 200's, every couple of minutes. It can be like morphine. I've known people go to the hospital with a fracture and they're popping *Arnica* and *Bryonia*, and people will refuse to X-ray them because they said, "You can't have a fracture because you're not in enough pain." They examine it and they want to send them away. I've seen that happen a couple of times with children. They say, "There's no way this kid's fractured." You have to really tell them, *"I demand an X-ray!"*
Audience: Do you give *Arnica* and *Bryonia* at the same time?
Ian: What I start doing is *Arnica* first, repeatedly, and then if the pain persists despite the *Arnica*, I look for a pain relief remedy. And *Bryonia*, I've found, is probably more often needed than any other single one in that situation. Especially if you get that "worse from the slightest movement," they just want to immobilise it, keep it completely still, any movement will aggravate it.

Same thing, those of you who are treating people with a so-called "slipped disc." Someone has a sudden jolt, their back goes out, or they have a fall on the back, something like that. If it's a fall, it's more likely *Hypericum*. But if someone's back suddenly goes out and they just can't move, you know, you see these people and they're being lifted onto a stretcher, every little movement is agony, that's *Bryonia*. That's the *Bryonia* situation. Better than *Arnica*. When you get into high potencies, usually it will work better.

Think of *Hepar* if they can't stand it being touched. So you try *Arnica*, because we know *Arnica* has that symptom, fears the doctor. They don't want to be approached or touched. A person in shock will often have that response, and *Arnica* can deal with it. But some people, it's that the area is so sensitive and so painful, and *Hepar* has that hypersensitivity more than *Arnica* even. So just the slightest touch, even just some clothing touching the area that's been affected is so painful - give them *Hepar*.

Audience: This is when you really learn what's characteristic of the remedy, when you see it in an acute.

Ian: Yes, exactly. And you really only need one thing that's very strong in the patient. You need to match that to a remedy that has it equally strong. It's not like you need a list of things.

One remedy that some of you may not have used in a situation like this is *Calendula*. *Calendula* is particularly good for compound fractures, and also, of course, anywhere there's an open wound or a laceration as well as a fracture, you need *Calendula*. *Calendula* is the great sepsis preventer, and it should be internal and external. I only ever used to use *Calendula* externally, as a lotion or an ointment, and then I learned about it as an internal remedy. It's a great remedy in potency. It's one of the best post-surgical remedies that I know.

Audience: Is your only clue to use *Calendula* the open wound. Are there any other aetiologies for it?

Ian: A lot of pain. It's interchangeable with *Hypericum*. So if someone has post-surgical pain or they have a lot of pain due to a fracture, for example, a wound of any kind, and if you try *Hypericum* and it doesn't work, use *Calendula*. I've sometimes seen it work much more effectively. With *Hypericum*, there needs to be nerve damage for it to work, or nerve trauma, whereas *Calendula*, it could be other times of pain. It could be soreness pain.

Another one that's in there that you might not think of for fractures is *Eupatorium-perfoliatum*. Many of you will know that as an influenza remedy, and the characteristic symptom is the bone pains. And the characteristic type of pain is that it feels as if they're broken. So, according to similars, that makes *Eupatorium* a good remedy for broken bones, right? Just like *Ledum* has a sensation as if a puncture wound, so it will heal puncture wounds. So *Eupatorium* will also help with bone pains. A person can rarely, when they're in an acute fracture situation, they can rarely say the pain is in the bone. It's like, "It hurts." That's when you need *Arnica* and these more general remedies. But once they've got it set and so on, if they've got a lot of pain in the bone itself, go to *Eupatorium*, and it will usually take that away pretty effectively. It's also one of the top remedies for bone cancer, to relieve the pains from that. As far as I'm aware, it won't do anything for the cancerous process. It doesn't have an affinity with that disease process, but because its affinity with the bone is so strong, it can relieve the pain.

Hypericum, you probably will be aware, the main affinity is with the spine, and the nerves in general. We know it as a nerve remedy, but in the context of bones, wherever the spine is involved, think of *Hypericum* as probably the first remedy. I wouldn't generally bother with *Arnica* first, if someone's fallen on their spine. The typical thing, someone goes down the stairs and they fall down every stair on the coccyx. This is painful, from what I remember. It's quite a painful thing to do. Anything that involves the spine first, switch affinities. Go to *Hypericum* first, and then give *Arnica* later, if you need to. There's not so much soft tissue there. Someone's fallen right on the coccyx, you need a nerve/coccyx remedy, and *Hypericum* is your top one. Also, if anyone's been injected, they may need *Hypericum* to deal with the effects of the injection. They're having an anaesthetic injection or something of that kind, a lumbar puncture, all those things, horrible things.

We've got two remedies that speed up the union of bones: *Calc.-phos.* and *Symphytum*. I personally find it hard to differentiate them. I don't know if any of you know of any particular keynotes. The only one I know that is a very good keynote for *Symphytum* is the pricking pains, if you get that. They describe it like a pricking sensation. These are people who've got a plaster cast and they want to get their fingers down there and itch it. It's like a pricking-itching.
Audience: It's interesting, because if you take a leaf of the plant, it's got all those little prickles.
Ian: Yes. *Comfrey.*
Audience: And if you wrap comfrey around a fracture, it will make it prickle.
Ian: So if you ever see that symptom, I'd go for *Symphytum* first. What I actually got into doing was giving them both together. I know you're not supposed to do this. But you know what? It works really well. So I would give something like *Sympthytum* 12c or 30c once a day, regularly, and then I'd give *Calc.-phos.* 6X as a tissue salt, three or four times a day, in addition. Those two together will work ninety-odd percent of the time. You can heal up a fracture very, very quickly. That's my approach if I can't figure out which works best, then I use both. They seem to complement each other.

Audience: I had a gentleman, an elderly gentleman that had very bowed legs, and they were doing surgery, and when they got in there, they decided they couldn't do the wedge that they had anticipated, so they split the bone longitudinally, and moved it over and did a whole lot of reconstruction there. He was in a hospital where they not only didn't believe in homeopathy, but the daughter had already asked, and they made a really big deal over it. So she carried everything and sat there by her Dad's bedside. She gave him pre-op, and afterwards some remedies. I told her, "No *Symphytum,* no *Calc.-phos.* until the doctor says everything's cool," and it's ready to just mend. The doctor came in the first day after the surgery, and he says, "Oh, my." And he called all the other residents. He called all the other surgeons, he said, "Seventeen years of surgery, I have never had a leg do this well! I wish I knew what I did differently!"

Question: Did you tell?

Audience: No, we couldn't. You have to get used to this not taking the credit, don't you? It keeps you humble. But what was beautiful, though, was that everything had gone so well that by the second day, he said the magic words that it looked like everything was lined up and looking good. He had X-rayed it again. So I said, "Now go to the *Symphytum.*" He never used another pain killer again. He had a drip he could push on demand. He never used it again. And he went home and did the *Calc.-phos.* and *Symphytum.* He was doing both. They said it was going to be three months because of his age before he would be able to walk on his leg and have the cast totally removed. It was all gone in six weeks.

Ian: That's great. I usually quote people, I usually say, "You should be able to reduce the healing time by at least a third." And that to me is a confident prognosis. If they have an expected healing time of three months, then with homeopathy it should be two, maximum, so six weeks is great. That's good going. It's like you've halved the time, actually. And that's not unreasonable. We should expect that. It's how it should be. You live and learn, don't you? So I find that combination works really well. Has anybody else had an experience of using them together?

Audience: I had a similar experience with a kitten that had a compound fracture of the pelvis. And the vet pinned him, did this procedure, and when it came time for the midpoint check-up visit, the assistant took me aside and said, "What have you been doing with this cat? The cats are usually in so much pain and so cantankerous by this point that we can't even handle them." And this cat was so happy and calm.

Ian: Right. It's like its so outside of what they're used to that it blows their mind. This is great. The great thing about first-aid is it's the only way that surgeons and allopaths are going to get *Arnica* experiences, when the patients go in there and demonstrate what homeopathy can do. And sooner or later, they'll get it. We can't tell them in a way that will convince someone who's never been exposed to it. The way I look at this, *Calc.-phos.* to me is nutritional in this context. It's as much nutritional as homeopathic. So I see the *Symphytum* as being the more the homeopathic remedy, stimulating the self-healing response. *Calc.-phos.* is feeding the tissues. That's the way I justify my polypharmacy in this context, not that I feel bad about it, but if someone has a problem with it, I can usually persuade him with that argument. It works really well.

There's one other remedy at the end there, which is the *Thyroidinum*. Some people have thyroid problems. That can cause poor bone recuperation. And some people, the bones will refuse to unite because they have a sluggish thyroid, usually an underactive thyroid gland, in which case you can use *Thyroidinum*. I would generally use that in a low potency, in the 6c or 6X, three times a day, as an organ support remedy. You'll see that written about in Clarke's *Prescriber* and Clarke's *Dictionary of Materia Medica*, and I've used it and it's been successful. So if in spite of the *Symphytum* and the *Calc.-phos.*, they go back and they say, "It hasn't set," and they can't understand why and you can't understand why, check the thyroid, and treat it, if necessary.

One other remedy that's useful to know is *Bovista*, and that's when the fracture itself has healed, but there's a lingering œdema in the joint, which I've spelled the English way. There's no "o's" in oedema. Is that the way you spell it? Oedema in the joint so that the fluid gets drawn to that place and stays there. Do you know what *Bovista* is? Puffball. That's what we call it. It's those things that if you prick them, they go boom, they go up in powder. Anywhere you see that there's kind of a puffy swelling, that you can push your finger into, think of the puffball, by affinities.
Audience: This is after?
Ian: Yes. You've treated the bruising and it's healed and so on, but the puffiness is still there.
Audience: Would you do the same thing for an injury that happened a long time ago and has caused further problems since?
Ian: One thing is, was it treated the last time? What I would generally do first is to treat it with the remedies that they should have been given at the time, because that is a "never well since" scenario. Something that seems to have healed, and then two years down the line, the ankle or whatever it is, suddenly flares up. I would give them the remedies that you would have given them at the time -

16

retrospective first aid remedies like *Arnica*, *Ruta*, or whatever seems to be indicated. If that doesn't work, then the chances are they need a constitutional remedy that has an affinity with that area, which we'll talk about later today. You need a bone, a joint, or whatever it is affinity constitutional. It could be a *Calcarea*, for example. If it's the back, it could be a *Kali*. They've all got affinities like that.

If that's the only thing that's gone, if there's nothing else wrong with the person, and suddenly their ankle's gone lame or it's swelling up, I would treat it as first-aid. Look at the picture, look at the modalities. If they've never had *Arnica*, give them *Arnica* first. And then they may need *Ruta* or *Rhus-tox.* or *Bryonia*.

Ruta is a good one. The main thing to bear in mind with *Ruta*, is when the lameness remains, everything's healed, but there's a feeling of weakness in the affected joint or limb. This is where I used to err on the side of under-prescribing and then I learned to do the opposite with traumatic problems. Because if you don't treat that remaining lameness, they're going to compensate for that, it's going to change, if it's a leg or it's a knee or something, it's going to change the way they walk, the way they stand, the way they sit, it can often throw the back out. You see a whole chain of health problems, because you didn't help clear up that last ten percent. Often the patient themselves, they're ninety percent better and they think, "I'll leave it now, it's O.K." But you really pay attention. Is that person walking normally? Can they do everything on that ankle that they could do before they injured it? And if they can't, keep treating, keep treating until it's well. Otherwise, they'll end up with a chronic health problem. And it's often a precursor to arthritis and stuff like this, because it's something that wasn't fully healed. Why is that funny (laughing)?

Pam: I was thinking of Oink (Danaan's cat). He has a cat that has a limp. This is a cat with a history of severe trauma.......
Danaan: By the way, another health tip for any open sore, infected sore, is honey. It'll cure those kind of problems. My cat - his arm was run over by a car and they were going to cut his arm off. It was infected and gangrenous. He was on antibiotics, he just had flesh, all the hair was gone, they kind of sewed him together. I just filled a condom with honey and put it over his arm every day for a week, and his whole arm grew back. Honey's amazing stuff.
Audience: But he's still limping - is it a bit shorter than the other?
Daanan: Well, he lost two toes, because they were gone, pretty much, but it saved his arm.

17

Rhus-tox. and Related Remedies

Audience: Is *Ruta* worse heat?

Ian: No, it's usually worse damp, if anything. The modalities of *Ruta* are almost identical to *Rhus-tox:* worse first movement, better when they limber up, worse in the damp, generally speaking, and also worse using it, worse over-exertion.

Audience: Will you talk about how to differentiate between *Ruta* and *Rhus-tox?*

Ian: Yes. One thing I want to do with you is, there's a group of remedies that all look a bit like *Rhus-tox*. Maybe we'll do that right now, because it's there. I've had loads of cases where you give *Rhus-tox,* and it looks like the clearest *Rhus-tox*. you've ever seen, and you give it, and it doesn't work. There's a few remedies like that, and *Rhus-tox*. is one of them, for me, so after a while you get creative and find all the other remedies that look like *Rhus*.

So let's do that. Take *Ruta*, first of all. The main thing that will help you differentiate these two, again, is knowing the affinity, because you can't differentiate them that easily on the symptoms. *Rhus-tox*. is worse cold damp; *Ruta*, it seems, is worse cold applications. Both will often respond to warmth. Both are worse from over-exertion, from lifting, from straining. So they have lots of things in common. You have to look and see what do they have that's different? The main thing is the affinity. With *Ruta*, the primary affinity is with tendons and cartilage and the periosteum, the covering of the bone. This is the primary affinity of *Ruta*. And also the joint capsules, the synovial capsule membrane, etc. With *Rhus-tox.*, the primary affinity is muscles, over and above everything else. Then it has a strong affinity with nerves, then it has an affinity with tendons, and it also has an affinity with skin and cellular tissues. *Rhus-tox*. is a big remedy in cellulitis. That's worth knowing if you've ever treated cellulitis.

Audience: Ligaments fall under *Ruta*, then?

Ian: Yes, tendons, cartilage, ligaments, all fall under *Ruta*. *Rhus* has an effect on these, but it's not primary for *Rhus*. What's primary for *Rhus* is muscles, whereas *Ruta* affects the muscles, but the primary affinity is with the tendons, cartilage, ligaments, and the periosteum. So, it's a question of trying to see where this pain or this problem is coming from. That's why affinities can help you when symptoms don't. So you can have a case that looks like *Rhus*, and you're giving it and it's not working, the chances are it's not a muscle problem, primarily. The chances are it's a tendon, or a ligament or a cartilage or something of that kind.

The other thing you'll see is that, in terms of muscular problems, if *Ruta* is needed, it tends to be the deep muscles. For example, the big muscles down in the back, supporting the pelvis, where someone's had a really bad sprain, or a really bad injury of some kind. If *Rhus* seems to help up to a point, and then it stops helping, *Ruta* will often complement it, because it seems to go a bit deeper. It's the same relationship as *Arnica* and *Bellis-perennis*. You know that one? So *Arnica* is all the soft tissues on the surface, but if the injury is more internal bruising, *Bellis* will follow on. It will take up the work where *Arnica* leaves off. So *Ruta* has the same relationship to *Rhus*.

Audience: I have an amazing *Bellis* story!

Ian: O.K. We'll come around to that. Does that answer your question of the difference between those two? The main difference is the affinities. One other thing, in terms of the symptoms. The strongest symptom that I look for to confirm *Rhus-tox.* is a sensation of stiffness. The idea with *Rhus* is that it's stiff, it's like the rusty gate. They want to loosen it up, it's a bit creaky at first, and once they get it moving, it's not so bad. That stiffness is probably the strongest characteristic, which is why they're worse first movement, better continued movement. It's something that needs limbering up. Once the muscles get warmed up, it's not so bad. Whereas *Ruta*, the strongest thing to look for is lameness or weakness, which is not the same. One is stiffness, the other is lameness or weakness. And a person will often go through, in their healing process, they'll often go through a stage of stiffness, where they need *Rhus-tox.* more than anything else, and then they'll be left with a stage of lameness, but this is usually afterwards. The relationship is usually that way around. It's usually *Rhus-tox.*, and then it's *Ruta*. *Rhus* will help up to a point, and then if it stops helping, *Ruta* will pick it up.

Now I'd just like to talk about a few other remedies that look like *Rhus*, because *Ruta* won't always finish the job off. One of the remedies that I found very, very useful - it looks like *Rhus* in many respects - is *Radium-bromide*. Again, it's got virtually the same affinities, but in addition, it's got a strong bone affinity. So it has the muscles, also the bones, and the joints and the skin. And it's got similar modalities to *Rhus-tox.* One of the strongest modalities for *Rad.-brom.*, is better for heat. So if you've got someone with deep muscle pain or joint ache, or back pain and you think that they should respond to *Rhus* and they're not responding, and all they want is something hot next to it, and as long as they get that, it's relieved, have a look at *Rad.-brom.*

And the other one that has that strongly, better for heat, is what?

Audience: *Mag.-phos.*

Ian: *Mag.-phos.*, right. So if that is the outstanding thing - I remember a guy, he had these terrible back pains. He put his back out, or something, and he found through going in a hot shower, that gave some relief, but it wasn't quite enough. So he went and sat on a hot water tank, which didn't have much insulation, it was so hot, he almost burnt himself. He had to sit with his back up against this copper cylinder, as it was really hot, and he said he had to keep cooling off, because it was burning his skin. As long as he sat there, he was totally relieved. That was *Rad.-brom.* It helped him. *Rhus-tox.* ameliorated, but it didn't take it away. *Rad.-brom.* cured him.

Audience: And that guy in the Sebastopol clinic might have benefited from *Rad.-brom.* as well?

Ian: Right. He had a hot pack?

Audience: Yes - a heating pad.

Ian: It depends to what extent it helped him. He may have just been doing that. It may not have actually been taking the pain away.

Audience: Oh, you could tell it was helping. He was like: "Don't take this away," it was like his safety blanket.

Another one that's got very similar modalities, it may surprise you, is *Lycopodium. Lycopodium,* is better heat, especially in the joints. Joint pains, worse first motion, better continued motion, better for heat. So sometimes you need to go from the particular to the general, especially if this is a patient who needs *Lycopodium* as a general remedy, then it may be that their local symptoms are the same as their constitutional. So *Lycopodium* will often help, especially the knee joints. Someone's got problems with the knees, and it's got *Rhus-tox.* modalities and *Rhus* doesn't cure it, have a look at *Lycopodium.* Especially, which side is it going to be?

Audience: Right.

Ian: Exactly. So if it's the right knee or right hip or right elbow or right shoulder, and it looks like *Rhus* and it's not working. Check out *Lycopodium.* Any questions?

Audience: Would you see spasming in *Rad.-brom.* the same way as in *Mag.-phos.?*

Ian: No, it's more akin to *Rhus-tox.* It's stiffness, and sore pain, bruised pain, that kind of thing. It's not the same kind of lightning-like pains and spasms that you see in *Mag.-phos.* I don't think it has as strong a nerve affinity. I've seen some good cases of rheumatism and arthritis where *Rad.-brom.* is the best remedy. Where I practice in England, it's a very radioactive environment. We've got the biggest nuclear power plant in England just about thirty miles up the coast, and they keep releasing these "safe" emissions into the environment, which are well within government accepted limits, so it causes no health risk whatsoever. Only every time they do it, everybody gets these weird diseases. And a lot of it is like a flu. They get a flu-like thing, people just get sick really quickly. It's like a mini-epidemic, and what a lot of them are left with are joint problems. It's like a lingering thing that doesn't clear up. They get low energy and joint symptoms. They get rheumatic symptoms in the joints, and *Rad.-brom.* just blows it away, most times. So there is the aetiology there as well.

Audience: Maybe we should try that - there's a lot of releases of supposed safe levels of tritium at Lawrence Labs., here in Berkeley.

Ian: It's everywhere. *Rad.-brom.* will clear a lot of stuff, even though it's not necessarily radium that's been released. It's similar enough to some other types of radiation.

Another one that has sometimes fooled me is *Pulsatilla*. That can be a surprising one. Again with the joints, it has similar modalities: worse first motion, better continued. One strong difference with *Pulsatilla* is that generally, it'd be worse for heat. So if you get a case that looks like *Rhus* in many respects, it's a joint problem or muscular, and they say it's better when they loosen it up, but it's worse for heat rather than better, take a look at *Pulsatilla*.

Audience: Does that mean local heat on the area?

Ian: Yes. Or just generally, it can be either.

Audience: So they may say they want to ice it?

Ian: Exactly. They may actually say it's better for ice. The other strong one there would be *Apis*. If the person says something cold really helps, usually you're down to a couple of remedies. The top one would be *Apis*, there. It's much, much better for cold.

Audience: Do you give high potency or low?

Ian: Well, it depends on the intensity of what you're treating. If it's a first-aid situation, I prefer the higher. If it's more of a chronic, long-standing thing, I would start with the low. It's just my own preference.

And there's another one here in this group, and that's *Tuberculinum*. It also, believe it or not, has virtually the same modalities as *Rhus-tox.* in joint problems. What *Tuberculinum* also has as a characteristic are the wandering joint pains. It's the knees, and then it's the shoulders, and then it's the elbows, and then it's the hips, and then it's the knees again. It's like you're chasing it around. Ever see that? *Tuberculinum*.

Audience: *Pulsatilla* can have that too.

Ian: Yes, they overlap. *Tuberculinum*, especially if you see that in children. It's variously diagnosed as growing pains, and rheumatism,

21

and arthritis, and arthralgia. They get about three diagnoses, because every time they get it diagnosed, it's somewhere else. You see *Tuberculinum* will nearly always cure that in kids.

Audience: It sounds like we're wandering from acute problems into chronic problems, so are we talking about a single remedy for a long time or treating acutely or what?

Ian: Well, the patient determines that more than we need to determine that. Obviously, the longer-standing the problem, the more long-term will be the treatment, as a general rule. And if it's a chronic history with multiple aetiologies and different symptom pictures, then it may need a series of remedies to get them there. What I'm talking about now is just like a mini-picture, which could be the whole picture, or it could be one in a series. Some people are layered in terms of their pathology. If you reach a point where what you're treating now primarily is a joint problem, that's the affinity, then you want a remedy that has that affinity. So you're in this group, generally speaking, plus a few other chronic remedies, the *Calcarea's* and so on. And that's the last one I was going to mention.

If *Rhus-tox.* is perfectly indicated and doesn't cure, have a look at *Calc.-carb. Calc.* is virtually identical in its modalities: worse damp, worse first motion, better continued, better heat. And *Calc.-carb.* is the main chronic remedy, it's the chronic complement of *Rhus-tox.* So if *Rhus* helps, but it doesn't cure, if the person says, "Yeah, it's great, can I have some more?" And you give him some more, and a month later, they say, "It's still good, can I have some more?" So, it's really helping them, but it's not going quite deep enough, then you want a complementary remedy. It's not that you're on the wrong remedy, it's just not quite deep enough. So the chances are, they'll be a *Calc.-carb.* constitution underneath. You've got a *Calc.-carb.* person with a *Rhus-tox.* problem. If that *Rhus-tox.* isn't curing it, go to *Calc.* And in fact, if I see that's the case, I would generally, as soon as *Rhus-tox.* has done it's job, I would follow it with *Calc.-carb.*, whether they need it or not. All the old homeopaths say that the best time to treat the constitution is when the person is just finished with an acute. So if you see that relationship there, I would just give it to them routinely. This will prevent a lot of complications from setting in.

Audience: I had a patient who I gave her *Calc.-carb.* constitutionally, and emotionally and energetically, she's really better, but her joints are bothering her more, so I gave her *Rhus-tox.* the last three visits, and she's happy.

Ian: She's happy, good. I like that. To me, that's appropriopathy. You've been appropriate to the demands of the patient, because sometimes we homeopaths, we get fixed on what we think the patient needs. They come back and they say, "I'm sleeping better, but when are you going to fix my knees?" And that's what they want, so we have to really learn to listen.

Audience: The mother of a friend of mine who's had a lot of pain, it sounded like *Rhus-tox.*, and then she mentioned that she always felt better with her arthritis when she ate *Tums* (antacid calcium carbonate), so I gave her *Calcarea-carbonica*, and she got all better. She found her own remedy.
Ian: That's great. People know what they need, huh? On some level, we all know what we need. So that was a slight distraction, but it was a good one.

In fact, there's one other that mimics *Rhus*, and that's *Calc.-fluor.*, especially with back pain. If you get strained backs and it's got *Rhus* modalities and it's not curing, have a look at *Calc.-fluor.* Again, it's like a deeper *Rhus-tox.*, in terms of the muscles of the back, especially.

Audience: Ian, how about teeth, is there a specific remedy?
Ian: Is there a specific problem you have in mind?
Audience: Well, like the bone receding, loose teeth, things like that, losing bone.
Ian: That's a constitutional thing as opposed to first-aid or traumatic. What you're looking at will be the syphilitic group of remedies, primarily. I would favour *Syphilinum* over *Medorrhinum* in that. For loose teeth, the main two remedies will be *Syphilinum* and *Calc.-fluor.* *Calc.-fluor.* alone will often cure that, actually, but you have to stay with it. They may have to take it for a few months before it will actually work. But feel free to do both: *Syphilinum* high, *Calc.-fluor.* tissue salts. *Calc.-fluor.* is a deeply syphilitic remedy. So it has that affinity really strongly.

Prescribing Nosodes

Audience: Ian, I feel really nervous about giving the nosodes without really good indications. What's your experience been with that?
Ian: Well, maybe you're asking the wrong person, but you did ask me, so I'm going to answer. I have no prejudice against the nosodes, shall we say. In other words, I don't treat them as a category you have to be super careful with or anything like that. I'm more with Burnett. Burnett's approach with the nosodes was that people need them for the same reasons as they need the other remedies - they

have symptoms and so on, plus *they have other indications as well* that require nosodes. In other words, more people need nosodes more often than any of the other remedies.

Audience: What about our instructors who talk about "rousing the miasm?"

Ian: Yeah, sure. I'll just answer this quickly. If you look at a case history. Say there's a top layer which is their pathology that they're presenting with. That's what the patient wants help with. And then maybe there's a constitutional remedy underneath that. And maybe the same remedy will help both of these, who knows? The patient's remedy may help the migraine headaches or it may not. They may need a different one. And underneath that, there's a miasmatic background which includes the family history, their medical history, anything that's happened during their life, and so on. Now the question is, "Is that miasmatic background influencing every other level now, or not?" If it is, the chances are you'll never cure on any of these other levels until they get that nosode. You'll palliate only. They'll be better for a while, and then they'll relapse. They'll say, "That remedy you gave me for my hay fever was wonderful. Can I have another, please. It's come back." Right. What that means is that the miasm wasn't addressed. The underlying tendency was never treated. This person may well need a nosode, even though it's not their remedy. Their remedy will be this other one.

You take a good constitutional case and you'll see all the modalities and so on will be *Calc.-carb.*, or *Silica*, or whatever it is. It's not going to be indicated on every level, but what they have is a tendency to......, a recurring tendency for something to come up under certain circumstances. That, for me, is quite enough to justify giving a nosode. You give it when the time is right to give it. Normally, what I would do is, you treat, based on what's indicated. When you get stuck in the treatment, this is called "obstacle to cure." One of the main obstacles to cure is the miasm. Hahnemann and everybody said that's when you treat it. How can you disagree with these people? Experience will teach you this, if you just try yourself. You try not giving the nosodes, and sooner or later, you come up against these blocks and you wonder why the person's not getting well.

Audience: I still worry about blowing people up.

Ian: Right. The only time that I've found that you may blow people up is if you give a nosode that's completely not indicated now. So, in other words, a classic example I can give you that I've done is, say it's a child and I take their case, and what they're presenting with is loads of catarrh, mucus, sinus trouble, maybe asthma, O.K.?

And they've got warts. Everything they're presenting is telling me they're sycotic. So let's say they need *Thuja*, or *Pulsatilla* or *Nat-sulph.* - a sycotic remedy. Then I look at their background and they used to have allergies and problems with milk and they're frightened of dogs, and everybody in the family died of T.B. So now I've got prejudiced. There's so much tubercular stuff. And I look at this child, and they've got long eyelashes and blue eyes, and they're thin and narrow-chested. There you go, it's *Tuberculinum*. What I'm doing here is ignoring what they're actually presenting.

Audience: Which is going to start screaming at you.....

Ian: Yes. So I'm getting prejudiced. And if I give that child *Tuberculinum*, it's out of order. It's a remedy they may need on some level, but it's out of sequence now. So what will happen in that case is that they'll do more of what they were already doing. They'll come back and the asthma's worse, they're full of catarrh, their behaviour's got wild. So they're screaming *Medorrhinum* at me now. I don't conclude from this that I did something bad, or that I'm a bad person, or that I should retire from homeopathy (laughter)! Whatever conclusion you draw is up to you. What I conclude is that they needed that remedy on some level, otherwise it would have done nothing. It had to be similar. It had to resonate to do anything at all. The second thing is, the timing wasn't right. O.K.?

So you put it on the back burner. You say, "I'll come back to this." And now I'll treat what I can see. You'll see it much more. They'll come back with the worst headache they ever had in their life or something of this kind. You'll think you've given them meningitis or something! It's O.K. Their vital force in its wisdom is saying, "Look here, Bozo. This is what you should have been treating." It's not a problem. It's about being willing to just be flexible enough to drop what you thought was the case and see what actually is the case. It's not what I thought it was. The ability to respond is the key thing, I think. We can never always get it right the first time. You get as close as you can get with your case analysis, and then you've got to give something to find out whether you're right or not. It's that willingness to just try it. And as long as you're willing to respond to what happens, it's really O.K. Homeopathy is so forgiving. It's so forgiving. People will come back to give you another chance. They'll come back to complain about what you did to them!

Audience: I tell my clients that my motto is, "I'm ready to be wrong at a moment's notice," to try to get them ready for the fact that I may well be.

Ian: Who are you trying to get ready for that fact? I prefer not to be prejudiced either way. It's equally O.K. to get it right first time, you know! That's good too. It's acceptable.

More on Calc-fluor.

Let me just say a few other things about *Calc.-fluor.* It's just in my mind. It's buzzing around. I knew a guy, and he ran virtually a whole practice, for a number of years at least, his practice was run on major nosodes, five nosodes and twelve tissue salts. That was the basis of it, and he had one of the busiest practices in England. And the way he was able to do that was he knew them really well. He knew the nosodes really well and he knew the tissue salts really well, and the beauty of the tissues salts is that you can quite happily combine them. So if one of them doesn't cover the whole picture, you just bring in another to fill in the blanks. You kind of mix and match the tissue salts. So virtually all of his patients would get nosodes and then they'd get a blend of tissue salts, and he was treating pathologies, cancers, heart diseases, unbelievable things, chronic arthritis, and getting people off all the drugs and stuff. Nosodes and tissue salts. Every now and again if he saw a clear constitutional, he'd give that too. But he said he wasn't that good on the constitutional prescribing, so he stuck with what he knew.

Calc.-fluor., it's an interesting one because it's got a strong bone affinity, but it also has affinity with the connective tissues, really strongly. Connective tissues. Everything that holds all our bits together. I envisage that this is why it helps when the teeth are loose. It helps to keep them in place. It's such a broad spectrum remedy, *Calc.-fluor.,* if you think about connective tissue. One of the useful things that I learned about it is hyper-mobility of the joints. You get these kids that are the star pupil at school because they can bend their elbow back, and no one else can do it. They can send their arm around and they can do all these weird yoga postures and stuff. That's *Calc.-fluor.* It's the best remedy for that. And the way in which that often presents as a pathology is spontaneous dislocations of any joint, whether it be hip, shoulder, anything at all. It's the number one remedy, *Calc.-fluor.* for spontaneous dislocations.

Case Management

Audience: Do you find if you're treating at this kind of level, will you find that it has an effect on their constitutional picture, or not significantly?

Ian: Only if they need it constitutionally.

Audience: But you don't find that you're changing things so that it makes it harder to zero in on the constitutional remedy?

Ian: No. No is the simple answer. I tend to treat what the person has a problem with. So if they're brought to me because they keep putting their hip out, then that's more of a problem to them than the fact that they may dream of fish now and again or, you know, something that's not really problematic.

Audience: Well, I know when I started constitutional treatment, I never would have dreamed of asking for help for the things that I really needed help with, because I didn't know that they were accessible with homeopathy.

Ian: Absolutely. What I've found is the best, the simplest way to get people to a point where they're asking for help on other levels, is to give them what they want first. You treat on the level the person is comfortable with and that they perceive homeopathy can help them with, initially. So if someone comes along with a hip problem, I want a hip remedy first. As soon as they get help with that, the chances are they will not only come back, but they'll tell a thousand other people too. If I over-rule that and I treat these other things, they'll often have a negative experience with homeopathy. I've never seen it be harmful to the patient.

Audience: It's that old thing, isn't it, of seeing where the energy is tied up?

Ian: Yes.

Audience: And if someone keeps putting their hip out and ending up in bed, and it's giving them all kinds of pain........

Ian: There can be all kinds of spin-offs from that. It can become an aetiology for other health problems. And until you remove that, it's like people living at poverty level who have trouble seeing the value of getting help on another level. You have to remove that first. It's like the case you described. The *Calc.-carb.* helped generally, but the person still has their chief complaint. That, to me, is like a red flag. Especially if that red flag gets worse when I give them their constitutional. What that says to me is that the constitutional remedy I gave them is a good remedy for eighty percent of them, right? That *Calc.-carb.* was good for eighty percent, but if twenty percent of them has a *Rhus-tox.* problem, that twenty percent will never be cured by *Calc.* They need

Rhus-tox. too. And if all I do is give them *Calc.*, every time they get *Calc.* and it puts more energy into their system, there's only one place that healing energy can go. It can only go into their pathology. That's where that healing energy is being directed right now. So you give a remedy that's close to the person but not close to the problem, the problem will get worse. Kent says this is an incurable patient. I say his mindset was incurable, because Kent's mindset was that you can't treat diseases. You have to treat patients. That was his fixed idea. That was a limitation in Kentian homeopathy, which is why he says cancer and all these things were incurable, T.B. is incurable, cancer is incurable. You step outside of Kentian homeopathy and they're eminently curable. You look at Burnett and Eizayaga and all these other homeopaths who don't think that way, they cure these things routinely. Why? Because they're willing to treat the twenty percent first, and *then* treat the underlying constitution.

Eizayaga clarified this for me better than anyone else. He said all you have to do is apply Hering's law of direction of cure. The main ingredient we have to pay attention to in Hering's law is the reverse direction. Ailments will get better in the reverse order to that which they developed in the first place. That's the main criteria that you know that someone is getting well. And we get return of old symptoms showing that the person is getting back to their healthier state. See, the person has constitutional things here, which sooner or later, through aetiologies and traumas and vaccines and drugs, now it's compounded into a localised health problem, O.K.? According to Hering's law, you have to start the treatment here (with the most recent problems). It's contrary to Hering's law to start the treatment here, treating the person first, or treating the miasm first, or anything else. According to Hering's law, you should start with the problem that's presenting. Once you've cured that, then you treat the things that caused the problem in the first place.

Audience: This means to me that so often in constitutional prescribing we're really flying in the face of that direction of Hering's law, because we're trying to find the most comprehensive healing and often going back and back....

Ian: We're treating *there,* when the person's energy is tied up *here* right now.

Audience: Well how about if you treat constitutionally, and then it comes up and it jams? I have a specific client I'm thinking about, which is somebody with *Rhus-tox.* and *Belladonna* alternating, and it led me to the *Calcarea*. And now they're in *Calcarea*, with a deeper history of cancer and tuberculosis, and everything's coming out, but there's a hip that got stuck.

Ian: The hip?

Audience: The hip is just not moving with the constitutional, so in that case, even though it started off here, and it led me deeper, it still comes back, so according to what you're saying, the direction of cure, all the energy is coming up, like, in terms of direction, but it's sort of like you have to retrace a little bit.

Ian: Yes. To me there's no contradiction there. It's not a linear thing. It's hard to represent this in two dimensions, but it's not a linear thing. People will zigzag towards their own cure, and we don't know which way they'll go. And very often, you'll find an old problem, which was never fully healed, once they've healed the things which they've presented, that old problem will reveal itself now, for what it was. Before, they had so much energy tied up in the migraines or something else, that the hip wasn't bothering them. Now they're sleeping better, their headaches are better, when are you going to fix this hip? It becomes an issue now because they've got the energy to deal with it. So that's not a problem, and usually it's an old symptom anyway, and that picture will clarify the closer you get to it. And also the more you ignore it, the clearer it'll get. That's what I find. So the more you prescribe around that, the more energy will go into it, if that's what needs addressing. So sooner or later, you'll focus right into it and you'll say, "O.K., what are the modalities of this?" With a bit of time and practice, you'll see that it gets clearer and clearer and clearer. They'll say, "It's my right hip, it's waking me at 3:00 in the morning, it's going down to my knee." What's the remedy? It's *Kali-carb.* And it may be that they need a general remedy, but it's very specific for that problem.

And the same thing can happen on emotional levels. The person's doing really well physically and so on, or they're doing well generally, and suddenly they come back in what seems to you like a *Staphysagria* state, or an *Ignatia* state. They've suddenly gotten into a real state about something, and this again can be a return of old symptoms in the direction of cure. It doesn't mean that the person's getting worse. They came in happy and then they come back an emotional wreck. It's usually a good sign! They've got the energy to deal with that now. So you ignore what you're doing and you treat what comes up. Be flexible.

Audience: Well sometimes, according to the training I'm in, it would be more along the lines of intercurrents, so you have your constitutional that's there - the underlying remedy. And then you unravel, you continue.......

Ian: Yes. It's true. The way you find out whether it's an intercurrent or not is, "Did they go back to it?" If they do well on a remedy for a while and they go off on a tangent, and you give a new remedy here, if then they go back and return to that original picture, then it was an intercurrent. However, if they go back to a different remedy at this point, it wasn't an intercurrent. It was a curative remedy, and it was probably a zig-zagging cure. You're zig-zagging that patient towards cure. This one took them part way, and this one took them part way, and now they're on to something else. Sometimes you think it was an intercurrent, but it turns out it wasn't. They're actually finished with that. And I try not to get too fixed on knowing what the person's remedy is, because we can be so sure that we've found the constitution, and yet once you start treating them, all kinds of stuff can come up. It's good to be willing to let go of that quite readily. And it's hard when you've done so much work figuring it out! We get attached to our decisions, you know?

Further Thoughts about Calc-fluor.....

A couple of other things about *Calc-fluor.* You keep distracting me, but you're not going to get away with it! I wanted to mention looseness of the teeth, hyper-mobility, spontaneous dislocations, and what was the other thing?

Audience: Exostoses.

Ian: Thank you. You're right. Bony growths and spurs, exostoses. If you don't know what else to do, or in addition to whatever else you're doing, *Calc.-fluor.* as a tissue salt is the top one for the bony spurs. It's also a good support remedy in varicose veins. What I mean by a support remedy is, you may have to give other things as well. As a tissue salt, it will generally help.

Audience: Does exostoses and bony growths include neuromas?

Ian: No. Wait. How do you define a neuroma?

Audience: A neuroma is a growth of the connective tissue lining.

Ian: It's not the bone itself, is it?

Audience: No.

Ian: But it may be that *Calc.-fluor.* would also help that. I would also think of *Ruta* and you've got another group of remedies there. But *Ruta*, because of the affinity with the connective tissue is very good. Also, we're looking at the sycotic remedies more than the syphilitic. And that, again, is the value of affinities. The bone affinity would lead you to syphilitics, and if it's a bony growth, you need a syphilitic remedy. If it's more a connective tissue growth or a soft tissue growth, it's a sycotic remedy. *Medorrhinum, Thuja, Staphysagria, Causticum.*

The other thing about *Calc.-fluor.*, it's a great remedy during pregnancy. Backache of pregnancy, I would advise *Calc-fluor.* along with *Bellis-perennis,* these would be my top two remedies. Backache during pregnancy, where it's purely a mechanical thing. The woman's getting heavy, and she's developing backache as a result of that, and / or varicose veins, and / or haemorrhoids, all of these things *Calc.-fluor.* will help.

And the other thing it's good for is it keeps things stretchy that should be stretchy. So it stops them from going hard. It stops things from hardening that need to be flexible, so it's perfect during pregnancy where there's going to be a lot of stretching of things that don't routinely get stretched that way. I found that women generally recover a great deal quicker if they've had a course of *Calc.-fluor.*, especially in the latter months, like from the sixth month on, and just keep them on it right through to the due date.

Audience: I work with people who train for contortion......

Ian: This would be a useful one for them, together with *Rhus.*, obviously, there's a tendency to strain things, and also *Ruta.* That would be one of the group. Definitely.

Audience: And when you say, give it to them, would that be more in the tissue salts realm?

Ian: I routinely use it in tissue salts, unless it's indicated generally. If the person seems to need it on every level, then use it like any other remedy, high potencies and so on. I generally use a 6X or a 12X.

Audience: What you just said about *Calc.-fluor.* in terms of stopping things from going hard that shouldn't go hard, that's exactly what a bone spur is. It's the calcification of the periosteum.

Ian: Right. And another tip with those is, don't be afraid to give the remedy for months. It takes months to grow these things, and it can take months to dissolve them. But they can be dissolved. And the other thing I recommend is to use castor oil externally, every morning, every night, and it has the same effect. It will dissolve things that are hardening. If you do the two things together, you'll reduce the healing time substantially.

Support Remedies

Audience: How come *Calc.-fluor.* works for hypo-mobility and hyper-mobility?

Ian: Good question. How come *Calc-fluor.* works for contradictory states? Its got, on the one hand, the kind of looseness of joints and the hyper-mobility, and on the other hand, it's got the hardening, the tumours and bone exostoses and so on. And I think that there are several ways I could answer that question, but I'll do it the short way. We were just talking about this on the break.

One of the advantages that herbal medicine has over homeopathy is that they have things called regulators. So they have a group of substances, tinctures, herbs and so on which neither stimulate nor subdue; they regulate, which means that they can do both, depending on the needs of the body. And I think the tissue salts have the same effect, personally, more than the homeopathics. So a tissue salt can do that. A good example, the easiest one that you'll know would be *Nat.-mur.*, which is, as you know, sodium chloride. So if you give sodium chloride as a tissue salt, it will regulate the salt balance, the fluid balance, in the body. If there's too much, it will drain it. If there's not enough, it will increase your thirst and redistribute it. And you don't have to decide which side of the coin the person needs. You just give the remedy and let it take care of it. I think homeopathics can do this to a certain extent, but I think it's more true with the very low potencies and the herbal remedies. The things that are more nutritional have more of an effect this way.

Similarly with *Avena-sativa*. Think of that as an herb for the nervous system. Someone can be completely shot to pieces with nervous exhaustion, it will lift them up. Someone can also be hyper and too nervy, and it will calm them. It will act like a mini-tranquilliser, and we don't have to decide. That's why the homeopaths can really benefit from knowing some herbal tinctures and some low potency tissue salts. They will broaden the range of things that you can do, and you don't have to remember loads of symptoms. You just get a sense of the range of action, the type of action, and the tissues that it acts upon, and then almost any problem in that area, in that arena, will be helped, not necessarily deeply cured on every level, but it will help them enough that you can get the cure going, or it will support the other things that you're doing.

We saw a case in the clinic, last week, it was in Sebastopol, and this woman came in. She'd had homeopathic treatment; she got castor oil to rub on some area that was painful, which had been suggested, and she also had been given some enzyme treatment or something to help with the digestion. So I was doing the follow-up and I said, "How are you doing?" And she said, "Those enzymes, brilliant, took the pain away really good" - she liked those. "And that castor oil, magic stuff, I used that and it took away all the inflammation". How about the homeopathics? "Oh, that thing with the coffee and waiting half an hour, yeah, I took it sometimes, but it was a real pain." It was really interesting to me to watch the patient's experience of taking homeopathy versus taking things like this, herbal supports, nutritional things, things we consider to be kind of inferior to homeopathy. From the patient's perspective, they were doing more for her than the homeopathic remedy, which she experienced as being a real pain.

Audience: But the thing is, if it changes the symptoms and you're prescribing on the symptoms, would you take the whole case so you know what the symptoms are, and then it starts regulating on a superficial level or a cellular level? That's the argument I've heard about tissue salts, that if you're trying to get an accurate prescription, it wouldn't be doing that superficial a thing, but it would be changing the symptoms.
Ian: Right. Hopefully for the better!
Audience: That's the argument I've heard and I would think how would you get a picture of what's actually going on with the patient, because it's temporarily palliating it?
Ian: Right. But you know what, if the patient's getting better, does it really matter? And the main criteria I use to tell whether the patient is getting better is, "What does the patient tell me, and how do they seem to be doing?" It's not whether I've found their deep constitutional or not. It's like, are they getting better or aren't they, according to my own yardstick and also the patient's experience. Very often, people will get better on these things, very, very often. They'll actually move towards cure.

People used that argument with me when I started using organ remedies, and I started writing and talking about organ supports. They said, well it's no good giving a remedy for the liver or for the kidneys because it will take away part of the totality, so you won't be able to find the remedy the person needs, right? Good theory. I decided to just try it anyway and see what happened. What I found happened more often, which was a surprise to me because I hadn't expected it - you know when the patient's got a general picture, and then they have an organ which is functioning so inefficiently that it's actually taking up most of their energy. So someone has very weak kidneys or a very weak heart. All that healing energy is directed here now. If I give a remedy to that organ, I feed the organ and strengthen it, so it's functioning as near to optimum as it can. What I observed is that energy which was tied up there is now available for the rest of the constitution, which meant in practice, they came up with a clearly indicated constitutional remedy. It was clearer than it was before! It wasn't less clear. So it was actually the opposite to what I was told.

If you haven't tried this, I recommend that you suspend your prejudice about it, or anything that you've been taught, because I was taught the same thing, and yet when I tried it, it never happened. It really never happened. In fact one of the things that I often found was an indication to me that a person needed an organ remedy was that I couldn't see a clearly indicated constitution. My reasoning for that now is that they didn't have the energy to put out a clear picture.

If you think about which patients you get where they have the best constitutional pictures, most homeopaths will say, "Children." So you say, "Why children?" and they'll say its because they've got more energy. O.K. So homeopaths will tell you that people with the best vitality put out the best pictures, so the sicker someone gets, the less chance you have of finding the constitutional remedy, or the harder it will get for you. And this is why you end up with seven pages of information, sixteen aetiologies, they're on ten different drugs, they've had surgery four times. You look at the family history and there's every disease you can think of, and you try to find one remedy that covers all that and you go crazy! Homeopaths do - sweating over the computer for days. Meanwhile, the patient's not getting better. So try and suspend what you've been taught and try it. Don't take my word for it, try it. That's all I ask of you, and then get back to me in a year, and you tell me whether the patient's got only palliated and it made the case difficult, or whether they actually thanked you for what you did. What I found in my own practice is that people came back and they said, "Give me some more of those drops. Never mind those pills. Give me some more of those drops." I'd say, "Well what about that dose I gave you in the office?" "Oh well, that didn't do anything. This tincture, I know, is working." And I learned just to listen, to listen to what people tell you.

Audience: I find if I'm giving somebody a related thing, like if I'm recommending vitamins or herbs, if you're really familiar with what you're recommending for them, you know what to expect. If I'm telling somebody to take B vitamins and they come back and they're sleeping better and their dreams are better, I know what to expect of

B vitamins, and if I've gotten the right constitutional, it's going to go way beyond that.

Ian: Yes. It's going to be out of the range of what that can do. Good point. And what I've also learned is that patients know that too, after a while. Patients can tell the difference. They can tell what a tincture is doing, what a tissue salt is doing, what a flower essence is doing, and what a constitutional does, and they'll come back and report to you. I trust that my patients know. It's the same with people on drugs. Homeopaths often say that it's hard to treat someone on drugs because it masks the symptoms and so on. It's not my experience. Patients know the difference between what the drug does for them and what the remedy you give does for them. So I rarely tell people to stop the drugs they're on. I say, "Carry on with what you're doing. You know what that does for you. It's obviously not curing you, otherwise you wouldn't be coming to see me." Right? So they know the limitations of what they're taking. If you give them something better than that, they'll feel the difference. So it's the same really. You give them something that helps, and then you build on that.

Just one last thing on that. I don't want to harp on about it, but you give anybody any kind of remedy, whether it's a tincture or whatever, they'll improve up to a point, and then they'll tell you when it's no longer helping. And at this point, you come in with their constitutional, and hopefully what will happen is, they'll start improving again. So you and they know the difference. This has reached it's cut-off point. Burnett wrote about this. He said, "Every remedy has a stop point of action." It will help up to a certain point, and then the patient will go beyond the range of what that remedy can do for them, at which point giving any more is counter-productive. And that's true for constitutionals, nosodes, tinctures, everything. We don't need to know when the stop point is. I've had people quite happily on mother tinctures for six months, a year, two years. You know, someone's had a transplant or something, they may need an organ support for the rest of their life. And that's O.K. Sooner or later, the person will come back and say, "It's done this much for me, now how about my energy, how about my sleep, you know, this isn't cured yet?" They come in with what's left. It's not so difficult. The more you do it, the easier it gets. That's what I find. The more you think about it, the harder it gets!

Recurrent Fractures & Uses of Tautopathy

I've put a note on your sheet there, "tendency to recurrent fractures." You see the *Calcium* salts in there. There's another one there, *Cortisone*. If someone's on steroids long term, one of the symptoms from that can be a tendency to fractures, and there's probably other drugs that do that too. Anybody know any others? I know that corticosteroids can have that effect. Chemotherapy also. It's so toxic it'll just about wipe everything, but bear that in mind. If someone has a history of long term corticosteroid abuse, whether it be for medicinal purposes, or even the anabolic steroids can have a similar effect, consider giving it as what's called a tautopathic prescription. You actually give the potentized drug back to that person, and that will often cure them where indicated remedies won't.

Audience: In a low potency?

Ian: I tend to start relatively low. I would start in the range of somewhere between 6c, 12c, 30c. And, depending on how they do on it, be prepared to work your way up. You know some people, they act as though it's a curative remedy for them, in which case I would stay with it, if they get a really good response.

Just one other tip on that, if you see anyone with joint problems, for example, and they've had injections - do they do that here? I'm sure they do, these cortisone injections into the hip, and also gold injections, these will often present an obstacle to cure. You've found a well indicated remedy which will help the person generally, but it will not help the area that was injected with cortisone. That's often what I've found. Remedies will just work around it, and it seems like it just gets numbed because of the cortisone. And so what I use is *Cortisone* in potency, whenever you see that that's the case. And I saw some amazing cures with it in fact, where nothing else was working, I would just give *Cortisone* 30 or 200, and it would actually cure the problem. It was like the only remaining problem was that it needed antidoting.

Audience: Would you give *Aurum* if somebody had gold?

Ian: Yeah, I've done that too - *Aurum-metallicum*.

Audience: What is tautopathy?

Ian: Tautopathy is the name given to potentizing the substance that has poisoned the person, basically. "Tauto" means "the same," so you're giving the same thing back to them that poisoned them. So if you have a child and they've never been well since the DPT vaccine, you give them *DPT* as a remedy, then that would be tautopathy. It's not truly homeopathy.

Audience: Is isopathy the same thing or something different?

Ian: It's very similar! It's almost the same, but not quite. You could read about this in that green book! I've done a whole chapter on each of these. Those terms have got a bit confused. What they're generally taken to mean is, tautopathy is things like drugs, vaccines or other poisons or toxins, things that the person has ingested, usually. If you give that back to them, we call it tautopathy. If it's more environmental things or allergens, that kind of thing that you give back to the person, we call that isopathy. "Iso" means "identical." "Tauto" means "same". It's very confusing. We would probably do well to create one new term that embraces both. The other time you would call it isopathy is when you're giving the same disease nosode for the disease that they have. So if someone has T.B. and you give them *Tuberculinum*, that's also isopathy. If someone has hay fever, and you give them *Mixed Pollens*, that's isopathy. They overlap. They're both useful and they'll both get you out of a fix quite often.

Audience: Have you ever given anyone coffee?

Ian: Coffee?

Audience: If they're addicted to caffeine and that's like an obstacle to cure?

Ian: Yes.

Audience: That would be a similar idea?

Ian: Yes - exactly. Or *Tabacum* if they're a smoker or *Chocolate* if they're hooked on chocolate, these kinds of things. The interesting thing is - you see, if it matches the symptoms, then it's homeopathy. If you're giving it purely on the basis of that's what they took and it poisoned them, then it's tautopathy. Homeopathy is the reason for giving something. It's very interesting to think about. The same substance can be homeopathic, it can be tautopathic, it can be herbal, it can be a tissue salt. It can be a combination of those things. Nothing is inherently homeopathic. It *becomes* homeopathic because it matches the state of the person.

One other remedy that I want to draw your attention to is *Syphilinum*. So if you work in a clinic over time and you hear about the fact that they fractured their hip or they sprained their ankle or something, and you treat it and fix it up, and then a year later, they're in with another one, and six months later, they've done their shoulder, and then you hear they're in a car accident. That tendency, you know, is part of the *Syphilinum* picture, and I've often missed that. You get so focused on treating the individual thing that sometimes you have to stand back and see the bigger picture. You say, "Hang on, a minute, they've got a tendency here."

I've got a colleague in England, and her son is about fourteen, and it seems like every time I hear something about him, he's broken something. So he's fractured this, and then he's done his knee, and then he's sprained his ankle, and then he broke his foot, and then something fell on his head, and of course she's treating all of these things individually, and well, and he's healing up really quickly and astonishing the surgeons and so on. But the fact is, he still keeps having them happen. I said to her, "Have you given him *Syphilinum?*" And she said, "No, why?" And I said, "Just look at his history for the last couple of years. He's had like seven or eight breakages or accidents of different kinds." That's *Syphilinum,* that tendency to keep doing that. And sometimes *Syphilinum* will also heal up lingering fractures and things that haven't healed on the other remedies. What the person's telling you is that the syphilitic miasm is an obstacle to the cure. That's why it's not healing up.

Audience: Would that be like a 1M potency you might give then?
Ian: Sure......
Audience: I want an answer!
Ian: Yes is the answer! I often give it like this: 30-200-1M. Three doses in twenty-four hours. This is the solution for indecision (laughter)! If you can't figure out which one, you give them all. It works really well.
Audience: What about the ones where they have the mixed potencies, say a 200X, and it contains everything in between?
Ian: I've really no experience with using it.
Audience: I haven't either, I just wondered.
Ian: I don't know. I'm sure they work fine. I wouldn't know when to use that as opposed to something else, but it's a similar idea. There seems to be a fashion for this more now, even among more classical homeopaths, to give a high potency one dose, and then to give a daily dose. It's become much more popular than it used to be, quite recently. They give a 1M and then a 12C once a day, or something of that kind.
Audience: They all do that at Hahnemann.
Ian: Vithoulkas developed this fashion, as far as I know. He got into using tissue salts and so on, mostly because people wanted something to take once a day, so he'd give them a daily dose as well. They have more credibility. It's like, "Is that it - *one pill?*" It seems a bit crazy. There's some anecdotal evidence that you can achieve more in less time. You can compress time a bit more.
Audience: I was just wondering, because one of the rationales that I've heard on the mixed potency is that the body takes the potency that it resonates with, and you don't have to deal with the guess work

of which potency is going to act best. I know two pharmacies that make them up that way.

Ian: It's a great theory, isn't it?

Audience: I don't know if it works.

Ian: There's only one way we can establish these things, and that is to test them out. It's the same reasoning that says if we have a combination remedy with ten remedies in it, the person will just take the ones they need, and ignore the rest. Who can tell? How can we measure that? The only criteria we have is, "Does it cure people effectively? Does it cure people as effectively or more effectively than giving single remedies, in single potency?" We have to test these things.

Scar Tissue

Let's move on a bit. I want to talk a little about scar tissue here. You see *Calc.-fluor.* coming in again there, a great dissolver of scar tissue. Anything that has *"Fluor"* in its name will have an affinity with scar tissue. The other main one there is *Fluoric-acid*, which is a good one for scars that kind of erupt. Rather than healing, they break out and they start itching and burning and become like an inflamed area.

Remember *Calendula* for open scars of any kind. I should put a few others in there.

Audience: What is proud flesh?

Ian: It kind of stands proud, it sticks out. It becomes a raised area, like a bump, something like that.

The main constitutional tendency to produce cheloid scars - anybody know what a cheloid scar is? Where you get an overgrowth of scarring. It's *Carcinosin*. So if you know that someone has that history and they're having surgery, or they get an injury or something, give them *Carcinosin*. You can do that virtually routinely. It's a very, very well confirmed indication. And you usually find a cancerous personal history or family history if there's a tendency toward cheloids.

Audience: It sounds more sycotic.

Ian: Overgrowth - yes. You have to perceive that cancer is the combination of the other miasmatic tendencies, so you've got the sycotic element, you've got syphilitic, and you've got tubercular. And then psora is the backdrop for all of these. Whenever you see *Carcinosin* indicated, you will always see indications for one or more or the other miasms, always. That confirms it. It doesn't mean they need a sycotic remedy rather than this one. What that may show you is the direction they took before they got towards cancer. So you'll often see indications for *Medorrhinum* or *Thuja* or *Staphysagria*. These are all great remedies to which *Carcinosin* is complementary. It means the person is coming the sycotic route. Another person, you'll see *Phosphorus*, *Tuberculinum* and *Silica*. That person's coming the tubercular route.

Audience: There's that saying about *Carcinosin*: "It's the marriage of all of the miasms, with *Alumina* as the best man."
Ian: *Alumina* as the best man? I've never heard that.
Audience: Third stage syphilis produces cheloid scars. Do we start with *Syphilinum*, then *Carcinosin*, or give *Carcinosin* first?
Ian: If the person has syphilis, and they're in the third stage of syphilis, and now they have a cheloid - is that what you're saying?
Audience: Yes, the third stage always has cheloids.....
Ian: The thing to determine is, "What needs treating the most now?" Is it the syphilis itself or is it just the cheloid. If it's just the cheloid, I would say, "Yes, the *Carcinosin*." But if they actually have active syphilis, and they have symptoms from that, then you would need a syphilitic remedy first, not necessarily *Syphilinum*. It could be *Mercurius*, *Phytolacca*, something of that kind, *Phosphorus*, *Arsenicum*, or one of the *Fluoricums*. They're all syphilitic.

Let's just touch on *Thiosiaminum*. It's very closely related to *Calc.-fluor*. It has the ability to dissolve things which have become hardened, especially scar tissue and adhesions. I wanted to especially draw your attention to its power over adhesions. It's the number one remedy for problems due to adhesions. This is typically post-surgical problems. If someone's had them out, and now they're getting pains and internal problems because of the adhesions, which will often result in more surgery. People get into a vicious cycle with this.

Radiation Burns

Audience: Could you please comment on radiation burns, leaving orange-peel skin afterwards on the breast tissue, and also post-chemotherapy where there's induration of the bladder, very common?
Ian: O.K. I'll comment briefly. The first one was breast tissue, it has like an orange-peel skin, so they're burnt from the radiation. The best one I know for this that I know is *Sol*. You know that one? Potentized sunlight. This is one of the remedies that get homeopaths the reputation of being a bit wacky. So I'd recommend *Sol*, like at

200C, that would be my first suggestion in a case like that, where someone's had radiation treatment and the appearance or feeling as if they'd been burnt. The next one I'd consider is *Causticum*. So if they have been burnt and never well since, you treat it like any other burn. *Causticum* will often take care of that.

There's also a flower essence which is very good for the ill-effects of over-radiation. There are several, actually, but one that I know that works very, very well from my own experience is called *Mulla Mulla*. It's an Australian plant. It's in the Australian Bush Flower Essences, and you can give that in drop form, and it will also take away ill-effects of radiation, especially if they're burnt. The easiest thing would be to try the *Sol* first. I've used that preventatively as well. Someone's having radiation, especially on the breast. The breasts are more sensitive to being burned, probably than any other tissue, so I would often use that routinely, give a dose of *Sol*, and it usually takes it all away. It's very, very good.

And your other question was what?
Audience: When the bladder has become hardened, and that's after chemotherapy, I know two people who are dealing with this. This is like nine years ago or six years ago, they had chemo, and the bladder is hard. They have recurrent infections. Would you look at *Calc.-fluor.* for that?
Ian: I would, but I'd look at the picture that's produced, the symptom picture that's manifesting. So they have recurrent urinary infections, and anything else with that?
Audience: The one woman has actual lesions. They've gone inside and looked and she's got all these little almost like ulcers, small, very small.
Ian: In the bladder?
Audience: And she's had multiple courses of antibiotics, of course, to try to control all of that.
Ian: Right. So, I'd probably be looking for a bladder affinity remedy, also.
Audience: I looked up *Merc.-cor.*, because it had ulcers in the bladder.
Ian: Uh huh. You see we have a rubric, *Induration of the Bladder*, and also *Induration of the Urethra*. The remedy that's listed under Induration is *Pareira*. You know that one? *Pareira brava*. It's a kidney and bladder remedy. So that's where I would start. I'd try to find a bladder affinity remedy that has that kind of problem. As a support measure, you could also use *Calc.-fluor.* tissue salt. Probably on its own, it wouldn't be enough.

Audience: Would you use *Equisetum?*

Ian: Yes. I mean, its the number one organ remedy, for the bladder - *Equisetum.*

Audience: As a support?

Ian: Yes. That would certainly strengthen the bladder and optimise its function. It may not cure the induration, but it would optimise the function, so you could try that as well, and it may well help.

Scar Tissue & Adhesions

Audience: Can we go back to *Thiosiaminum?*

Ian: Yes, I was going to.

Audience: I wanted to ask you, I think I have a case where it would help somebody. This lady's had three back surgeries, and we've been doing acupuncture on it, and it takes away her back pain, but now she has more pain in the adhesions from all the surgeries.

Ian: That's the one.

Audience: I gave her *Thiosiaminum* 30C once a day for three or four days and waited a couple of weeks, and nothing happened.

Ian: Right.

Audience: Should I have given her a different potency or something?

Ian: Well, sometimes I've found that just changing the potency will make the difference between it working and not working. When I first started using it to dissolve scars and so on, I was using like a 6X or a 12X daily, and over time it would work. What I found was, people who had a lot of pain, particularly abdominal pain, or whatever, following surgery, and I tried the 12X, it often didn't work. What I learned was that the 200C often did, so sometimes it's just a potency issue.

Audience: How much 200, how often?

Ian: Just give a single dose, and then give the person a packet and say, "You repeat it when you need it." Let the patient decide. They take a dose, and as long as they feel relieved, they don't repeat it. If they're better for six hours, then they repeat it in six hours; if they're better for three weeks, then they repeat in three weeks. I let the patient decide. And usually they should need less of it over time. So they might need to take a course of it for a few weeks, and then they should be able to wean themselves off it.

I learned that from Foubister. Have you heard of Donald Foubister? He was a Scottish homeopath, and he worked in post-surgical wards and so on, and so he experimented with all of these things and he found that the high potency would often relieve the acute pain, whereas the low potency didn't. The low potency is good for dissolving something that's just thick and indurated, or whatever. If that didn't work, I'd consider *Carcinosin* for the patient, depending on whether you see any confirmation for it. That would be good, in the background. But I would certainly consider that. The tendency to keep having adhesions is also sometimes part of the cancer miasm picture. You could look at the case with that in mind. If there was anything else in the case that suggested that, personal history, family history and so on, I would give that. It's good to have a backup.

Audience: Wouldn't Castor oil be good for that too?

Ian: Yes, absolutely. Castor oil rubbed into scar tissues, even if it's an internal adhesion problem, have the person either rub it into the area, or better still, use a pack. If they get in a lot of pain, have them put the Castor oil on there and use a hot pack or a heating pad or a hot water bottle. You're absolutely right. That will often do better than a remedy.

Audience: I found St. John's Wort is good for that.

Ian: As an herb or as an oil?

Audience: As an oil.. It can be very good for pain and a lot of stuff. *Hypericum* oil.

Ian: I just want to draw your attention to *Silica*. If someone has a scar following a fracture, or after surgery or an injury of some kind, and then they have a scar, and then they get a disease in the old scar, in the site of the scar, the main remedy for that is *Silica*. So if they then develop an ulcer or an abscess or a fistula, and it's in the scar where they previously had surgery or they've had something which had healed up, but it's left a weakness, *Silica* is the best remedy for that. Even if they grow cysts or tumours or growths or something of that kind, and you perceive it's in the site of a previous scar. You see a woman who has breast cancer, and she has it removed, she has a breast removed, and then it recurs in the site of the scar, *Silica* would be the top remedy, and *Graphites* would be the second. So you should be able to do a lot with scars.

There are certain local things like that which are very amenable to homeopathic treatment. Really, if someone has a problem like that, it doesn't matter what their constitution is. You may just have to treat it very directly to get a result. A remedy like *Thios.*- I've never seen a *Thios.* constitution in my life! I don't expect I ever will. It's a local remedy.

Audience: There's a case......

Ian: Oh God, someone's found one!

Audience: All local remedies. There are three cases in one of the

43

proceedings from the Seattle conference. There were three cases of *Thiosiaminum*. They were all specific, local problems. It worked beautifully.

Ian: O.K. So they haven't found all the delusions of *Thios.*, and all the dreams, and all this stuff?

Audience: They have some mentals....

Ian: Did it cure them?

Audience: I don't remember.

Ian: That would be interesting.

The thing is, sometimes - in fact quite often, I reckon - if they have a local problem, they can put out mental symptoms which are secondary to that local problem. It's not that they have primary mental symptoms. The mentals are secondary to this, so what they need is a remedy to cure this local physical disease, and when you cure that, you take all those mentals with it. If you treat cancer, for example, you'll see that over and over and over again. Since they have the bone cancer, now they've got despair and depression and anxiety about health and fear of death, all these mentals. You could repertorize those mentals for days and not find a remedy which cures the patient. It's very interesting.

Audience: Chronic conditions, though, will often give rise to irritability......

Ian: Yes, pain of any kind will do that. If you put someone in pain, it will bring out mentals which they didn't have or experience before. You could still say they were of that person, which is true, but they're only experiencing it secondary to this physical problem. Therefore, where do you aim your remedy? Here, (the local disease) primarily. You have to treat the problem. You can use the mentals to help differentiate the remedy, but don't just give the remedy for the mentals. And don't use it as the primary reason for prescribing either. The person has a physical disease. It's a mistake I've made so many times.

Muscles & Nerves

Let's move on a bit. We're going to move on and look at some muscle and nerve affinity remedies. I'm not attempting to do all of them. I'm attempting mostly to do ones that I'm familiar with and the commonly indicated ones, and I'll just mention a few of the smaller ones, rather than overwhelm you with lots of little details.

I've kind of mixed these in together, muscles and nerves, for no particular reason. Some of the remedies have both, have the dual affinity, like *Rhus-tox.* is both muscles and nerves. *Ignatia* is another example. So we'll just run through these ones. If you've got any questions, feel free to ask.

So we've got *Bryonia* in there, first of all. The kinds of pain that a person tells you they're experiencing is often diagnostic of the type of tissue that's affected. I'll say that again. The type of pain, the type of *sensation* that the person is describing will often help you in diagnosing what tissues or what disease process they actually have, if you learn sensations. So if someone has, for example, a sharp stitching pain, and they have it in the chest, quite commonly that will correspond to a pleural membrane type of pain. For example, if someone has pleurisy, or they're recovering from pleurisy, it's characteristic of pleurisy to get that type of pain, to get that stitch. And *Bryonia* is such a good remedy in pleurisy because it has the affinity with the lungs and it has that type of pain, as does *Kali.-carb.* - lungs affinity with stitching pain. So when you combine the two together, the sensation with the affinity, you've got a much stronger chance of finding a good remedy for the person.

But we also get sharp pains in the muscles, and this is where *Bryonia* can come in for muscular problems. It's very, very complementary to *Rhus-tox. Bryonia* and *Rhus-tox.* are like two sides of one coin. Dorothy Shepherd - do you know Dorothy Shepherd? She wrote good books: *Magic of the Minimum Dose, More Magic of the Minimum Dose, A Physician's Posy,* and, that was it, I think. She found from her own experience treating fractures, rheumatism, joint problems, arthritis, that very often the person would do really well on *Bryonia* for a week or so, and then they'd need *Rhus-tox.* for a week, and then they'd need *Bryonia,* and she couldn't find one remedy that covered both. And so what she ended up doing was alternating them. So they take *Bryonia* in the morning, *Rhus* in the afternoon, *Bryonia* in the early evening, *Rhus* before bed, and so on, so they'd get a dose of each, or two doses of each, every day. They're very complementary, so I personally have also done that, and you can do more in less time by combining those two.

The interesting thing is that they have opposite modalities of course: *Rhus-tox.* is better for movement, *Bryonia's* better for keeping still, and yet sometimes, a patient will tell you that they're better for movement and they're better for keeping still, or they're worse for movement and they're worse if they keep still. Some patients I've seen, they can't differentiate. They say, "It hurts if I'm lying in bed, and it hurts if I get up and move." So you think, well, which one is it?

Audience: Or, "I'm feeling restless, but it hurts when I move."

Ian: It's like, well, is that *Rhus* or is it *Bryonia?* Some people do seem to have mixed modalities, so in these cases, I don't sweat over it too much. I tend to give both in alternation, and then I let the patient decide which one helps them best. And usually after a few days they can tell you. They can feed it back to you.

The next important one is *Causticum,* which has got a really strong affinity with the muscles and also what we call the fibrous tissues, the cartilage and so on, the connective tissue and the tendons. Two key things to look for with *Causticum:* one is a loss of strength, when the person is losing the ability to do the things they can normally do with that limb, and the second thing is the contracture. So whenever you see that contracture is occurring, *Causticum* should be the number one remedy that jumps into your mind. Contracture - you see a tightening, a shortening, and a drawing in, whether it be a whole limb, or a single muscle or a finger or whatever it is. Contracture, think *Causticum.* There are only two other remedies that I think of where contracture is probably as strong as it is with *Causticum.* They would be *Guaiacum,* which also has stiffness and contracture as its strong keynote, and the other one is *Formica,* which is made from those little creatures that are everywhere at the moment. What is it?

Audience: Ants. It's the ant. So the venom from the ant also produces contracture and stiffness. So it you see that it's a strong feature, usually it will be in that group: *Guaiacum, Formica* or *Causticum.*

Audience: How do you distinguish them?

Ian: It's a good question (laughing). I don't know! The modalities are a bit different. In *Causticum,* usually, locally, they're better for warmth. So if it's a joint problem, they're usually better for warmth. Generally, they're usually better for damp conditions, which is unusual in joint pains. If someone is rheumatic and so on, the majority that I've seen will say that damp is worse rather than better. So if you ever see that peculiar modality that they actually feel better when it's damp or wet or raining, *Causticum* is probably your top remedy. *Nux -vomica* would be a close second.

The other thing with *Guaiacum,* the strongest thing you'll see there is it's worse heat, better cold.

Audience: Is that one of the small joint remedies?

Ian: Yes, you could characterise it as that. So that's the main modality you could look for, which helps differentiate it from *Causticum,* better cold applications. And *Formica,* I don't know in terms of main modality.

Audience: *Plumbum* also has contracture and weakness.

Ian: Yes, it does. We should add it to the group, add it to your list. Thank you. You're right. I've given *Causticum* to cases where I should have given *Plumbum*. It's a remedy that I've often missed. *Plumbum* has that combination of weakness - it's the main one where you get foot drop or wrist drop, so it's very often localised to just one foot, one hand, something of that kind.

Audience: Speaking of contractures, I've had this question about seizures, epilepsy and so forth - is that primarily psoric? Is that considered psoric or not?

Ian: I wouldn't say so. I would say, probably, if you wanted to categorise it miasmatically, true epilepsy, I would say is more tubercular. But having said that, it's such a broad thing that you could make a case for virtually any miasm, but if you think of the top remedies, you'd probably find more tubercular affinity than any other single group. Of course you'll find psoric remedies there too.

Audience: I had a good book on miasms, and I couldn't find seizures clearly listed under any of the miasms.

Ian: Right. I would say, true epilepsy, usually you'll see tubercular is the strongest history. If you're treating someone now who has epilepsy, the family history, usually, what I see, is more tubercular.

Audience: Or someone who has developed seizures as a result of a blow to the head?

Ian: Well, how do you categorise that?

Audience: I mean that happens quite frequently.

Ian: Well, that, you could say is psoric. It's more like an environmental, external thing.

Audience: It's also just traumatic.

Ian: Yes. General trauma.

Audience: You wouldn't say a broken leg........

Ian: I don't know. Does it help to categorise these things miasmatically? Not always. It's not always helpful. But I mean, seizures since a bang on the head is very amenable to homeopathy, and also from emotional shock, very amenable, whereas what you might call idiopathic epilepsy is much harder to treat.

Audience: So often when there's a head injury and there are brain wave changes or seizures after, they get anti-seizure or barbiturate drugs for years for this.

Ian: And then they have poor liver function as a result of the drugs.

Audience: Depression is a major side effect of those drugs.

Audience: Right. I have such a case now, which is why I'm trying to look at seizure.

Ian: It's very treatable. You need to look at a step-by-step approach. If the main thing that presents to you now - some of those cases that I've seen, by the time they come to you, they're just like a zombie.

The life energy is gone, the vitality, there's a mask-like expression, there's a flattening of the emotions, there's often constipation, there's a slowness, there are skin symptoms, and all of that is from the drugs, so you can't get near treating the constitution or the disease until you treat the drug layer.

Audience: And this person had this during most of their hormonal shifts, puberty, adolescence.

Ian: Right, so I'd just start with what's presenting, and start with a detox., and if you can, reduce the amount of drugging at the beginning of the treatment. Often a liver support will help more than anything else at the outset of the treatment. And all those drugs, the barbiturates and so on, are toxic to the liver. And you'll see that the depression and irritability are all liver side effects. Constipation, and all that stuff. So if you didn't know what else to do, do liver support, and it will give them enough energy to put out some symptoms, and it will start to detoxify them also. The other thing you can do is *Nux-vom.* and *Sulphur* in alternation. I see we've talked a lot about alternations today. There you go, *Nux-vomica* 6X and *Sulphur* 6X, alternated. Two doses of each daily, and do that for about ten days to two weeks. It's a very good detox. routine for people who've been heavily drugged. So you give one of them first thing, and the other one mid-morning and the other mid-afternoon, and then last thing, just alternate, so they get two doses of each.

Audience: Would you ever tend to whip them up too much though?

Ian: What do you mean, "whip them up?"

Audience: You know, an aggravation, but more like a confusing?

Ian: I haven't seen that. What I have seen is elimination on this.

Audience: But because it's 6X, it's more. . .

Ian: No, it's because they need to eliminate.

Audience: Is it manageable? I guess that's what I want to know.

Ian: Oh yes, absolutely.

Audience: Because you know how sometimes people will detox. and it's excessive.

Ian: The way that it's manageable is that you can always reduce the dosage, the frequency. If they're taking two a day, you can cut it down to once a day.

{While the tape was being turned over, someone commented about a person they knew who had some kind of profuse elimination using *Nux* and *Sulph*.......}

Ian: Right. That tells you how toxic the person is. You see rapid elimination on this. That's the idea. So if you tell the person that may happen, you may get diarrhoea, you may sweat, its not a problem.

Audience: Not everyone wants their insides on the outside.

Ian: This is what homeopaths tell other people is O.K., but when it happens to them, they don't like it!

Audience: Can you do this while the person is still taking their medications?

Ian: Yes.

Audience: So this just basically gets rid of the accumulation.

Ian: Exactly. It's that whole historical stuff they will tend to eliminate very, very quickly. These are both liver and bowel support remedies, so that's what seems to get stimulated, more than anything. The liver will get stimulated and the colon will get stimulated, so people will often have rapid bowel movements and they'll often sweat, and you may see signs of liver detox., like headaches and so on, and a furred tongue.

Audience: Is the idea of detox. that you can use it for anything that needs detoxing or is that kind of drug-specific?

Ian: I know it more as drug specific but, you know, drugs and chemicals, things that the person has ingested over time, and they're just kind of awash with something.

Audience: So you wouldn't use it for something that's just kind of like a chronically sluggish liver so they're all backed up?

Ian: Oh, yes. I do. Which is a lot of people.

Audience: Most people in our society could use drug and alcohol detox.

Ian: Exactly. What I found was that more people were *impressed* that something dramatic happened than complained about it, you know. It's only the homeopaths that wince when they aggravate. Most of the patients, they're like, "Wow, that's powerful stuff!" They like it, they really feel like something's working. You can always give them permission to cut it down if it's too much. The other time where I find this really effective is if the person is on multiple drugs of different types. They're taking Valium to make them sleep, they're taking uppers to get them up, they're taking painkillers every day, they're taking hormones, and you think, "Where the hell do I start?" And it's really hard to try to treat a case like that when they're so toxic, and so what I do is I start with a detox. routine, and then try to eliminate the drugs that they really don't need, or get rid of the ones that they can happily dispense with from the beginning, and then you treat on the picture that comes up. You'll see a much clearer picture within a fortnight.

Audience: So that particular thing is something you've done with a lot of people?

Ian: Yes. Lots!

Audience: It sounds so marvellously simple.

Ian: It's a routine thing. And I learned it off someone who had used it for fifteen years, who in turn learned it off someone who had used it for thirty years. I didn't make this up. This was taught to me by someone who had tried lots of other things and they found that this one really works.

Audience: So you might think of using this as opposed to *Chelidonium?*

Ian: Yes. This is more general. It's kind of broad spectrum, if you like. *Chelidonium* is specifically liver, when you're sure that there's liver weakness, they've had a history of things that weakened the liver definitely, whereas this one is more general, so they could be on nerve toxic drugs as well, or hormones as well, or contraceptive pills, it's more for a range of things.

Audience: A history of drug use?

Ian: Yes, tons of antibiotics, that kind of stuff, so the bowel function is all to pot, as well as the liver being weak.

Audience: You would use this for anti-psychotic drugs as well, Prozac?

Ian: Yes. And the effect of it is that it cleans the windows so you can see what you're looking at. It doesn't do anything to the constitution, unless one of these (*Nux* or *Sulph*) happens to be their constitutional remedy, which is possible, but not that likely. But what it does, it cleans the windows, and it will put energy into the system. I usually get them to report in about a week to ten days, so it's quick. You don't send them away for three months! You say, "I want to hear from you within about ten days." Usually I give a ten day course and then assess. If they do really well on it, I keep them on it for longer, give them another ten days on it. Most people within the space of two or three weeks, they'll clear what it can clear at that point. You can always come back to it again if they seem to get plugged up again.

Audience: If somebody is already on a constitutional that may be working, will that knock it out?

Ian: If someone's already on a constitutional and it's working, why do anything else?

Audience: Well maybe it's not working very well (laughter). Well, no, I'm thinking of a particular person, and he's really hard to work with and he's got a toxic history, and anything that happens with him is going to be very, very slow.

Ian: The thing is, if you can see a clearly indicated constitutional, give it. Don't complicate it. This is more for cases where you can't see that because of the drugs, because of the toxicity, like the case Jane was describing where they're on these barbiturates and now they're all drugged and they're all dopey, and you don't know which symptoms are the patient's and which symptoms are the drug's. That's a better case to use this. If you take a case that's clear *Pulsatilla*, give *Pulsatilla*. Don't mess around. And it will work. If you can see a clear picture, it will work, most times. This is more for when you can't really see the wood for the trees.

Audience: In this case, they've had *Sulphur* in high potency for several years, and their depression lifted for a little while, and then it didn't any more, and I'm thinking maybe there's some level of detox. that they need.

Ian: Maybe. Again, the question is, "Is there an indicated picture or not?" If you can see a clearly indicated remedy now, forget this. Go with what they're presenting. This is more when you really can't see it or when everything you give seems to bounce off.

Audience: Is that like lack of reaction?

Ian: Yes. This is lack of reaction. It's lack of reaction, or it's what you might call a one-sided case, where half of the picture just isn't there. They haven't got the energy to put it out. Or they can't remember!

Audience: So with this, you would get some kind of movement, whereas if you actually prescribe on a one-sided picture, the patient's unhappy.

Ian: Yes.

Audience: Because the way I've been trained would be you would wait and get more symptoms, but technically, this is a very nice way to get more symptoms.

Ian: I'll tell you, it's a darn sight quicker! And there are these cases that, it's not that we don't have enough, but that what we have isn't crisp enough. It isn't well enough defined to say, "This is this remedy." It's a bit of this and bit of that and it's all very kind of vague. A lot of people are like that, and it's because of the toxicity as much as anything else.

There are all kinds of other things that you can use to help detox. people. You can use algae, blue-green algae.......

Audience: I know someone who uses a dilute solution of bleach. He said only a certain kind of bleach works......

Audience: I was going to use it (*Nux* and *Sulph*) myself and ask if this would be the case. All the mercury in my teeth - I was being very affected by it, I had chronic fatigue, etc., so I had it all taken out. Every once in a while, under stress or exhaustion, or whatever, the symptoms will kind of come back. I can't get rid of them, no matter what constitutional remedies I take. I can't take *Mercury* as a remedy. Would this be a case where this might help to detox. from that sort of thing?

Ian: Probably, yes. And what it does is it stimulates the liver, colon and skin.

Audience: Could have some nasty results?

Ian: But it's effective.

Often the reason the body is having a problem is that its trying to put it out somewhere else, in the glands or the mucus membrane, or somewhere like that. And it's not working. So what it stimulates are the natural channels of elimination, which would be the colon, the skin, the sweat, the liver. I like it. I've used it many, many, many times and very rarely seen people have such a strong reaction that they couldn't handle it. And if that happens, I just cut it down. I've had a few people where their skin's broken out really powerfully within days. I've had people who've sweated buckets overnight as soon as they started taking it. And the nice thing is it's not even their constitutional. It's not that well indicated! Anyway, I don't know how you got me on to that, but lets just do a few more things on here and then we're almost at lunch time.

I put *Coffea* on there. I think *Coffea* is an under-prescribed remedy generally, probably even more so in American culture than in English. We're the tea addicts, but coffee is such a big part of the culture here, and coffee is a nerve stimulant. One of the things that coffee produces is a person who's running on adrenaline, someone who's stretched to the limit. They're using adrenaline energy to keep going rather than real energy.

When a person is stretched to the limit, a little extra thing seems like a big deal. And that's why you see with *Coffea*, if they're in pain, everybody knows about it. If they have a toothache or a backache or a spasm or something of this kind, it's a big deal if someone's in a *Coffea* state, because it's like the last straw. They were on the edge anyway and every little thing pushes them over. So the main thing to look for with *Coffea* is someone who's in pain and they can't stand it, the fact that they're in pain. Two remedies there: *Coffea* and chamomile is the other one, *Chamomilla*. And you'll see that *Chamomilla* is listed as an antidote to *Coffea*, and I think, vice versa. If you try one and it doesn't work, try the other.

But it's a good one for nerve pain, neuralgia of all kinds, including toothache. I put *Gelsemium* in there which has a very strong affinity with muscles and nerves. And you've got the loss of power, similar to *Causticum*, but *Gelsemium* is much more short term. *Causticum* is someone who's gradually declining, someone who's developing a chronic disease state. *Gelsemium* is more recent onset, and it's often through, for example influenza, or through a period of overstudy, or through anticipation of some ordeal.

The main thing with *Gelsemium* is that they're so weak that they tremble; they get the shakes, so you can often diagnose this one just by looking at the person. They get weak-kneed. You know what it means to be weak-kneed? Something's coming up and you're anticipating it and you're a bit nervous, and you get the shakes. I've seen a lot of people with problems with the knees, and the thing that they have is that they think the knees will give way. You see that? That can be for different reasons. *Gelsemium* is one of the remedies that has that, especially when they're going downstairs or downhill. They have to hang on to something. If that results from an injury, it would be *Ruta*. If someone has a weakness in the knee following an old injury or a cartilage operation, or something of that kind, it would be *Ruta*. We'll talk more about that this afternoon.

And the other one that has that weakness in the knee, if it's more arthritic, think of *Kali-carb.*, especially if it's the right side. The best characteristic of *Kali-carb.* is that they have the feeling that the knee, or the hip, is going to give way. It generally doesn't, but they feel as if it will give way, that it's not going to support them.

I put plenty of notes in there on *Hypericum*, for those of you not familiar with *Hypericum*. It's the best nerve trauma remedy that we have, especially the spinal injuries. I put another one in there, *Ignatia*. I stumbled on that one by accident, for people where their back suddenly goes into spasm, and no one knows what's wrong, and they don't know what's wrong. And it's variously diagnosed as slipped disc and other things., which it isn't. And they have osteopathy and it doesn't make any difference. This is very often emotional trauma that goes straight into the muscles and the nerves. And because they've internalised it in that way, they and you won't be aware that there's any emotional trauma. It's like you won't see someone in any emotional state, because it's gone straight into the body. What you'll see is someone who's in a lot of pain and spasm. Where I found *Ignatia* very, very good is sudden spasm and sudden paralysis. Somebody *suddenly* loses the use of a limb or something of that kind. I remember a ten year old boy who couldn't get out of bed one morning, couldn't use his legs, and it's several weeks later, and he still can't move his legs. And they couldn't diagnose what was wrong, and they were giving him all these nerve tests, and they think he's got some weird kind of neuropathy, and so on and so forth.

We took his case, and it transpired that the day before it happened, his parents had decided to separate. So it's like the boy overhears the conversation, his parents decide to separate, he goes to bed, and the next morning he can't move his legs. It's his way of keeping them together for a while, I think, unconsciously. So that emotional trauma went straight to his nervous system, paralysed his limbs. We gave him *Ignatia* 10M, and the next day, he came back to life. It was all removed, and he was able to grieve, talk about it, or whatever he needed to do. So it can be pretty dramatic, *Ignatia*. It can look like a serious disease, but it isn't. It's emotion that's gone straight into the body.

Audience: This is like hysterical?
Ian: Yes. You see it in the books described as that.
Audience: It's somaticized.
Ian: Somaticized, yes. So this is true psychosomatic illness. I think that we assume that more stuff is psychosomatic than actually is, personally. I think a lot of things go the other way. Or they just happen together. You know, a person has an emotional state and a bodily thing which corresponds. It's not always true that one *caused* the other, but in this case, it is.

I also put *Kalmia* in there. It's one that you may not be that familiar with. A very big neuralgic remedy, *Kalmia-latifolia*. It's got a heart affinity as well as nerves. So some people with heart pathology will do well on *Kalmia*, where they get the typical pains going down the left arm into the fingers, with numbness. But they can have these types of pains anywhere, shooting around. And it's got a particular affinity for the ulnar nerve, pains going down through the wrist and the hand, into the fingers, especially the third and the fourth. Very painful. Someone that needs *Kalmia* would be in a lot of pain.
Audience: The pain needs to be there? Not just ordinary neuralgia?
Ian: Oh, you could try it, yes. But usually with *Kalmia* it's sudden, quite painful, and then it's quickly gone. They come really fast and it really hurts a lot, and then it's gone again. If it's more like a lingering thing and it's there all the time, it's probably not this one. You'd be looking at another remedy. *Mag.-phos.* similarly has pains which come on fast and they're very intense, and they go fast, better for heat. I find that if you put *Mag.-phos.* in hot water it often works quicker than if they take it on the tongue. So dissolve it in hot water. Tissue salts are perfect for that. They're quick dissolving. They can just sip it as they need it.

I'm going to talk a bit more about *Ruta* this afternoon. Any questions on those, muscles and nerves? Anything I missed out?
Audience: Is there a good book you'd recommend on tissue salts?

Ian: Yes. There's one by Boericke and Dewey which is pretty good. It's called *The Twelve Tissue Salts of Schuessler.* You know the one? That's probably the most comprehensive, and it's got cases in it and also it's got materia medica and therapeutics. It's quite old but it's all still good information. I've got another good one, but it's less comprehensive. It's by Chapman. It's a similar type, *The Twelve Tissue Salts*, or something like that, by Chapman. I learned just about everything I got from that one.

If no-one has any further questions, we're going to move right on and talk about a few specific conditions......

Audience: May I promote this book just before you get started? If anyone doesn't have this book, I highly recommend it. Those of you who do have it will know what I am speaking of. The title is *A Guide to the Methodologies of Homeopathy* by Ian Watson. It's small, compact, succinct. It's a juicy little book!
Ian: I should take these quotes down. These will go in the next edition (laughing).

General Therapeutics

I wanted to look at some specific conditions like sciatica, Raynaud's syndrome, bursitis, tendonitis, teno-synovitis and any others that come to mind, carpal-tunnel syndrome, this kind of thing. I'm just going to give you some hints and some things to have that you could at least try while you're figuring out what they need, and at least give you a sense of what the main remedies are. Some of these, you'll find a whole group of remedies and you need to differentiate. But usually there's one or two remedies which are like the leaders, and if you don't know what else to do, you could at least give the person that one, while you're thinking about it. That's my approach.

Raynaud's Syndrome

Let's just have a look at Raynaud's disease. It's not strictly musculo-skeletal, but I thought I would stick it in anyway, Raynaud's Syndrome. It's more of a circulatory disorder really, I guess. Quite common, certainly in England. Is it common here?
Audience: Yes. It's common in Oregon.
Ian: Colder climate, yes, I guess that's going to be true. Generally, for those of you not familiar, the symptoms affect the fingers, suddenly getting very cold, very white, and sometimes completely dead, a

lack of sensation. Often, people will get it while they're driving or some activity that involves holding onto something. I've seen people in England where, for example, they work on the roads. I remember a guy who was a pneumatic drill operator and he had really bad Raynaud's and that was partly the causation, working outdoors, cold weather. There's a group of remedies that we have that seem to work particularly well. I've seen *Natrum-mur.* be very frequently helpful in that condition. It's often a good remedy for people with cold extremities, even if it's a warm blooded person generally. They won't necessarily complain of being a chilly individual, but they often have poor circulation in their extremities.

Another one that has the symptom very strongly, especially if it's very painful is *Agaricus*. That's made from a poisonous mushroom. This one is especially good if it's painful and it's to do with cold, being out in the cold. It's one of the main remedies for frostbite. So people get out and they get chilled and then they get frostbite in the extremities. It would be a good remedy for mountaineers, mountain climbers and so forth, anybody who's going to Everest, or whatever the American equivalent is. You've probably got some cold peaks here, Colorado and areas like that, or people who are doing snow activities, working out in the snow. *Agaricus* should be in a kit for a person like that. I've seen it work pretty well.

Another one that's quite common is *Sepia*. Sometimes you see Raynaud's disease develop secondary to hormonal changes. Sometimes it comes along with menopause or it comes as a sequelae of pregnancy. "Ever since pregnancy, I've had this tendency. . ." So there's been a hormonal change, and that affects the circulatory system, and now there's Raynaud's syndrome. *Sepia* would be a top remedy there. And a close second would be *Kali-carb*. A good indication for *Kali-carb.* is when a person wakes up and whichever side they've been sleeping on, the fingers of that hand, or even the whole hand and arm, will be asleep. You know that sensation when you wake up, it's all numb? So if they sleep on the left side, they wake up and the left hand and arm will all be dead. If it's the right, it will be the right arm. *Kali-carb.* will usually help that.

Audience: That's a frequent complaint I get, but another one I get is that when they're lying on their left side, their right, the contra-lateral side goes to sleep. Do you know what the remedy is?
Ian: Yes - what's the remedy for that one, where it's the opposite side to the side lain on? Anybody want to guess? I can have a guess at that. One that I know I'm pretty sure has that is *Pulsatilla*. It has like

the opposite to what you'd expect. It's part of the nature of *Pulsatilla*, right? *Pulsatilla*, they can have relief from pain lying on the opposite side, but they can also have things aggravated on the opposite side. You can find that in the repertory, I think. It's not changeability, it's a general, *Sides, Pains go to the Side Lain On, Pains Go to the Side Not Lain on. Ignatia* and *Rhus-tox.*, he (Murphy) lists. Two we've already talked about. There's a few others there. He puts *Pulsatilla* in *Pains Go to Side Lain On*. Huh? Maybe I got it wrong.

Audience: Years ago I had this man come in with his right arm paralysed. He woke up that morning. He was drunk the night before, came home, fell asleep on his front porch, lay on the arm all night and damaged the nerve. I tried to cure him on *Hypericum* and he never came back. What should I have used?
Ian: I don't know. I would have tried *Nux-vomica*.
Audience: Because of the aetiology?
Ian: Yes, and the affinity. See, *Nux-vomica* is one of the top remedies for paralysis and nerve problems, plus it has the aetiology of drunkenness, so I would have a look at that. I would also have a look at *Cocculus*, ailments from getting drunk.
Audience: It wasn't so much the drunkenness as the way he laid on his arm all night.
Ian: You think it was a purely mechanical thing?
Audience: Oh yeah, because he was drunk enough so that when he slept, he didn't move around. He just stayed in one position for twelve hours, and pressed on the nerve for the whole twelve hours, so there was nerve damage.
Ian: Right. It was a pretty dramatic response!
Audience: It's happened to other people.
Ian: He would have had to have a predisposition for that to happen.
Audience: The doctor said that it happens to drunks often.
Ian: Really?
Audience: Yeah. They damage their nerves because they don't move. Plus alcohol is a nerve damager anyway.
Ian: I would say the alcoholism is part of that.

It just brought to mind a remedy that I read about in Clarke *(Dictionary of Materia Medica)*. It could be completely irrelevant but it's interesting. It's called *Piscidia*. *Piscidia* is a fish-killer. It's some poison that people used to put in the sea or the river and it would stun the fish. It would kind of paralyse them and they would float to the surface so that they could catch them. There's a great story in Clarke's *Dictionary* where some homeopath decides to have a go with this stuff and see what it's like, so he took a swig of it, and the next day, he woke up and his arm was in this position. And it's like, he hadn't moved a muscle in something like twelve hours. Who knows? It's probably not what the guy needed, but it's an interesting story.

I would look at things like "*sudden paralysis,*" *Nux, Ignatia, Causticum.* They'd be in the nerve affinity group, and then try to match that to the aetiology. See, *Hypericum,* what would need to be there would be a trauma, something whacking the person or an injury of some kind or a wound. That's probably why the *Hypericum* didn't work. This was more like immobility, wasn't it, that brought it on? I don't know what else to suggest.

Another one for Raynaud's is *Silica. Silica,* you'll usually see, if the person constitutionally needs *Silica,* that they're a chilly individual, the circulation is poor, the vitality is generally a bit poor, and so it's part of a more general picture. The person, themselves, will say they're chilly, they feel the cold, and they get cold extremities. But I've seen *Silica* cure it.

There's also one of the bowel nosodes that works sometimes when the other remedies don't. You all know about the bowel nosodes? These are a small group of remedies developed initially by Edward Bach, who went on to develop the Bach flower remedies. He spent the bigger part of his career fiddling around in stool cultures for about twenty years. So he was fermenting stool cultures and identifying the different bacteria that were found in the colon. And having done that, he gave it all up and went and plucked flowers for ten years. You can well understand! So there's one of them called *Proteus,* and it's got a very, very strong circulatory affinity, and it's a leading remedy in Raynaud's syndrome. It looks a lot like *Natrummur.* If you get someone who looks constitutionally *Nat.-mur.* and yet there's areas that the *Nat.-mur.* doesn't help. I've seen it cure migraine headaches in patients that I was sure needed *Nat.-mur.,* especially where they have things that come on suddenly and violently. So you've got a combination of say *Nat.-mur.* and *Belladonna* in a patient. They get these sudden terrific headaches out of nowhere, and they feel like their head's going to blow off, or something like that. Or they get sudden epilepsy or convulsions, or they get sudden paralysis.
Audience: And you wouldn't think *Glonoinum?*
Ian: Well, maybe *Glonoinum* would help in the acutes, but this is more for the underlying tendency, they keep coming on. And it's also the number one remedy for intermittent claudication. Who can describe intermittent claudication?

Audience: You walk and you take a few steps, and you can't walk any more because your arteries in your legs are hurting, using up. .
.
Ian: Yes. Is it a constriction or is it just a cramping or what?
Audience: A vaso-spasm.
Ian: Vaso-spasm, so it's like a spasm of the artery itself, or the veins or whatever, the blood vessels. So this is the number one remedy for that, that I know of, *Proteus*, where you see that condition.
Audience*: Proteus* is also a common bacteria that grows out in like nursing home tables, kind of a sepsis.
Ian: It's probably not the same, because Bach invented these names, and some of them have been used in other contexts. It may be related, but it's unlikely. It's an interesting remedy. Another little keynote for *Proteus*, if you don't know the remedy, is people who've had the experience that they've been living in a war zone. They've been living in a situation where there was a fear of death, for example, for a prolonged time, so there's often adrenal exhaustion as well. Like people who've been living in Bosnia or somewhere like that for the last few years, you know, like you could be bombed any minute, or you could get shot when you go out in the street, that kind of situation where there's a high tension, high anxiety environment. But for some people that could simply be their home environment. There's a potential for violence in the home, and the person's lived with that for a long time.
Audience: Or as if, someone who was a kid under that and is still living that way?
Ian: Exactly. They're no longer in the situation, but it still feels to them like that's the case, that they're under threat. *Proteus* is one of the best remedies. It's really interesting.
Audience: But it's one of the few remedies which is sold by prescription only at Hahnemann Pharmacy.
Ian: You need a special license to get this remedy?
Audience: Do you prescribe this the same as you would any other remedy, or do you use it like a tissue salt?
Ian: No, more like when they're indicated as a general remedy. But also the thing with the bowel nosodes, they're a bit like the standard nosodes. Each one of them has say five or six remedies within them, so if you see indications for two or three of these polycrests, and no single one of them is quite doing the job, then a bowel nosode will often do the job. So, the nosode *Morgan* is one of the bowel nosodes, and if you see indications for *Sulphur* and *Graphites* and for *Calcarea* all in the same patient, and you can't figure out which, you can give them *Morgan*. It's like broad-spectrum homeopathy.
Audience: And isn't there a whole repertory on MacRepertory™, of

the bowel nosodes?

Ian: Not on the bowel nosodes I don't think. Or maybe there is - I haven't seen it.

Audience: Here it is.......

Ian: O.K. There are also materia medicas on it. The writings were by Bach and Paterson, and there's quite a good Indian booklet by Dr. Gupta. He's done a compilation of the bowel nosodes that is quite good. There's only about seven of them, so it's not a great deal to learn.

So those would be my top remedies in Raynaud's: *Agaricus, Nat. mur., Silica, Sepia, Proteus.* There will be others. Individual cases will need others, but I've probably had more success with those than any others.

Audience: They're not necessarily going to have an Agaricus frame of mind?

Ian: No, no. Praying in front of mushrooms and things like that, there's not much call for that in the Lake District. It's nice if they're a bit twitchy. Sometimes I've used it just more as an acute, *Agaricus.* It's one that people hold, and so, if they're working outdoors and they can feel the tingling start and they can feel it's coming on, they take a dose and it will just stop it. So it may not necessarily cure the tendency in those cases. It's working like an acute remedy, in which case they'll need an underlying remedy as well.

Another really good thing for people with Raynaud's is to get them doing chi kung exercises. Get them doing finger rolls, this kind of thing so it will bring the chi into the fingers. It's very good. One involves the flicking outwards. You actually flick the fingers one at a time, and the other is more of a rolling action. You roll them individually out and then back in again.

Audience: I guess this is a version of a question I've asked at every seminar you've given.....

Ian: You like to get it in (laughing)...... that's consistency.

Audience: If you successfully cured the Raynaud's, and now they have a brain tumour.........you know the argument that the symptom is the body's best way of isolating and limiting the problem to the most expendable part of the body, and if you cure an acute, you run the risk of taking away a channel from the body that it needed to eliminate, so it goes to a deeper organ, what about that? The patient comes in and says, "I want my Raynaud's cured, this is driving me nuts," so........

Ian: I'm open to any possibilities, so for me, it's quite possible that the rest of the person is actually fine, for the most part, and that they have a relatively localised problem, which affects the circulation and manifests in the fingers, and apart from that, they're actually reasonably healthy. I don't assume that the rest of them is therefore constitutionally sick. Even though everything is connected to everything else, it doesn't necessarily mean to me that they're sick on every level. They may just have a local problem. How do I know if that's the case? Well, if I treat them locally and all that happens is that goes away, and the patient remains well, I'm happy and they're happy. And that happens many, many, many times.

You know, a child comes in and they've got a verruca on the foot and I give them *Thuja* 200, the verruca goes away, nothing else happened, nothing else changed. The rest of them was actually all right. That was all that they were manifesting at this time, so there's no problem with that, and you can help a lot of people with local problems.

Audience: Because the vital force does successfully limit the problem.

Ian: And that was it, that was the extent of it. Now there are other cases, of course, where this is, if you like, a small piece of a bigger jigsaw. And it's actually connected to things elsewhere.

Audience: Like oedema of the hand....

Ian: Yes, for example, and maybe that oedema is secondary to kidney weakness or something that's more generalised. Now, if that's the case and all you do is remove the local expression, and you don't treat what it's connected to, then sooner or later, the vital force will show you. And generally speaking, in treating the local problem, the patient will show you if there was something more general. In other words, they'll come back with it. They'll say, "Well, that was good, but what about this?" And the way I see that, it's the same as with the organs. If their energy is no longer tied up in this, that energy is available for healing on a deeper level now. I'm O.K. with that, either way. If they come back well, I'm happy. If they come back and say, "This is bothering me more now," that's also O.K. with me, because it was there anyway, and now they've revealed it to me. And what I've found is that they're much more likely to come back and give me an opportunity to treat these things if I treat the problem area first, if I give them relief in the problem area. So it's O.K. Sometimes I've seen that.

I remember a case where I treated a woman. She had a problem with her knee, and that seemed like all she had, and I gave her *Ruta*, and it took it away. A few months later, she came back and told me she was fine, and I believed her. And then she went off and she was out walking and she was going over a stile, we call them, you know,

61

going over a wall. She climbed over and she felt the knee go again. She phones me up, I look at the case, *Ruta*. I gave her *Ruta* again, only this time it didn't cure. So this can be a sign for you that what you thought was local is in fact more general. One thing is that it comes back again fairly soon. The other thing is that when it comes back, the local treatment doesn't work the second time. It's not holding. So what she's telling me is, "It's part of a greater totality."

And in her case, the remedy she needed was *Natrum-mur*. I got her in and took a fuller case, and there was actually a *Nat.-mur.* picture, one part of which was that she had fluid on the knee. *Nat.-mur.* has fluid problems, just as *Ruta* has local fluid problems. So I gave her *Nat.-mur.* and it completely cured it. And *she* was better. But both results were O.K. The initial *Ruta* was good. That's what made her come back the second time - the fact that *Ruta* had worked. As far as she was concerned, *Ruta* had worked.

Audience: And you kept getting more information on her as you went along?

Ian: Yes. So I try not to have any fixed conclusion about which is true and which is good or bad, or better or worse. Just treat on what presents and then, according to what comes back, treat again, or don't treat again. It's O.K. either way.

And remember the onion analogy which I'm sure you were taught in college. Chronic treatment is very often like peeling an onion. It's layers. All you can see when you first look at an onion is the outer skin. You can't see what's behind until you take that off. The only time you get to see it is when you remove the outer skin. That's the only way in which you can see if there was something beyond that or not, is to take it away. So how can you say there's something wrong with that? You don't get any permission to treat deeper until you treat superficial sometimes. A lot of it is to do with the patient's permission. I feel quite strongly that they give us permission to work in a certain area, up to a certain level, at a certain time. And only when that's been addressed is the person ready to move on to other levels. It's relatively unusual that a person comes in and they give you their deepest truth or their deepest fear or their deepest delusion about themselves at the first visit. It's very rare. It's nice when it happens, but I couldn't run a practice depending on that happening every time. It would narrow it down. Most people I'd be discharging uncured. I'd say, "I'm sorry, I can't help you, I don't know what your core issue is," which is what a lot of the classical homeopaths do. Or they beat themselves up for not finding the core issue remedy! Not a good idea.

Repetitive Strain Injury

Do you ever get "housemaid's knee" here? Do people have that? Gardener's knee? Ailments from working on the knees. Carpet-layer's knee, that kind of thing. These are structural, mechanical ailments brought on by occupation, and you can't just say to the person, "The reason you got that is because of your job. Quit your job." It's not helpful. You may need to give them some exercise or regimen that helps prevent it coming back, but also we've got to treat people with these problems. We're looking at remedies with the strongest affinity with the knee, and *Ruta* is one of the strongest, so we'll talk a bit about *Ruta*.

Ruta-grav., as well as the ligaments, cartilage and tendons, it's got a big affinity with the joint capsules, and it has as an aetiology of overuse of the part. And if a person has only overused a part, then they'll only have a problem in the part, at least initially. They're not going to have a generalised disease first off. This is a classic repetitive strain injury scenario, and *Ruta* is the number one remedy for this, where a person is doing a repeated similar thing with one limb, or one hand, or one joint, or whatever it is. Succussing homeopathic bottles every day is enough to give someone inflammation of the elbow.........has it ever happened in Hahnemann?
Audience: Nooo.
Ian: You've got machines to do it now, huh?
Audience: No, we've got a big mallet!
Ian: A big mallet?
Audience: The remedy fits inside of it. You strain something else, but it's better.
Ian: That kind of idea - someone's typing all day, something of this kind. The number one remedy for this stuff is *Ruta*, and it's also the main remedy for synovitus and teno-synovitus, where the synovial membrane and the tendons connected to it are all inflamed. Ruta can help this even if it's long, long standing. I've seen cases where they've had it as a recurring problem for two or three years. And again, I would often start out by doing constitutional treatment, and the patient in general would respond, but they would still have the knee problem. Bear in mind that people can get stuck in things which where at one time a simple first-aid thing. But because it wasn't treated as such at the time, it's now a chronic thing. It's part of their chronic picture. So they still need that first-aid remedy. *Arnica* can be a chronic remedy. *Ruta* can be a chronic remedy. Someone's never been well since they injured that knee.

Audience: Would you give a low potency?

Ian: I would tend to start lower with a 6c or a 12c, repeating it daily, two or three times a day. You can always go up from there. If it's a long standing thing and it's not too acute. When it's something that's kind of grumbling and recurring, it's a weak area, I would tend to use the low potencies repeated over a time period. Usually I'd start with a 6C or a 12C and I'd be giving that two or three times a day, initially for a period of weeks, and keep them on it as long as they benefit. With time they should be able to reduce it and stop.

Audience: If a person tears a ligament, does that actually heal?

Ian: They can heal, yes. They don't always heal perfectly, but they can heal, and they can be nasty injuries. And you would need other remedies alongside that. When they had first done it, you would probably need *Arnica*, initially, and some *Rhus-tox.*, and then *Ruta* would come in as the main remedy, usually, because of the affinity. *Ruta* would be the long-term restorative remedy. But people can heal these things, even things that are supposed to be impossible to heal can be healed. I've seen that. And people who've had cartilage operations several times. You know, they've had bits of the knee cap removed, and they've been told, "You'll never do that again," and with long-term homeopathic treatment, they've done it again, and it's been fine. Whether they've regrown it or not, I don't know. I'm open to that possibility. I also get people to use *Ruta* externally in these long-standing chronic things. So you get *Ruta* ointment or gel, and you get them to apply it every morning and every night. It's very, very good. It's basically the herbal tincture in an ointment base.

You know, people are using sound therapy now to regrow things that are supposed to be impossible to regrow. Pam has a tape recording of a woman who's interviewed, and she developed this sound therapy where she can hear which note your body is lacking. Have you heard about this? If you speak, this woman has a certain type of hearing. She's got this unique kind of hearing. She can hear which note is missing in your voice. So what she does is she gives it back to you, and all kinds of spontaneous healings took place when she did this. And they found it could cure autism, Down's syndrome, all kinds of things, a complete reversal. Her own son smashed his patella. It was completely mashed. There was about twenty percent of it left, and he had surgery and stuff, and they said, "No way can we do anything more with this, nor can anything else," so she started doing this sound therapy. She would make a certain tone and aim it at his body on a daily basis, and within about six months, he's got eighty percent growth back. It's supposed to be impossible. Nerves growing back and everything.

Audience: Is she in the States?

Ian: Yes. There's some amazing stuff around. People are developing these techniques, and sound therapy, this was the medicine of the Egyptians. They used sound, light, color and castor oil. All of these things are coming back now. All the ancient, ancient therapies. We think it's new stuff. You read the Egyptian stuff, and that was the fundamental basis of their therapy: sound and light and colour and castor oil.

Audience: Sound therapy is actually a specialty now.

Ian: Yeah. There are different branches of it opening up now, people specialising in certain areas. There's a French guy by the name of Tomatis, I think it is, and he discovered a correlation between sound and autism. He made the observation that a lot of children who are diagnosed autistic are actually hyper-sensitive to certain frequencies of sound. They freak out when you have the vacuum cleaner on or certain kinds of music. He found that this was common in children with autism. So what he discovered was that there were certain frequencies that they couldn't receive and others that they were more sensitive to and he took certain kinds of music and he basically re-frequenced it and played it to them. So it was like Baroque music with certain frequencies taken out and others emphasised, so it sounds like a mess if you hear it. But to people in this condition, it sounds wonderful. What they do, they sit these kids with the headphones on, they give them a half-hour, and they watch this child's face go, like their expression will change. This is someone who's been completely shut off for six years or something, and within a half-hour, they'd start responding, and after a couple of sessions, they're normal. Total reversal of autism, supposedly incurable. So he has a clinic in France and there are people in England doing this now, with a very high success rate. Amazing stuff, huh? Simple, non-invasive, non-toxic, incredible.

The other thing to think about with *Ruta* - it's a good remedy for ganglions and growths, growths which are coming out of the tendons or fibrous tissue. The classic is on the wrist, ganglion of the wrist. *Ruta* is the number one remedy. The second would be *Calc.-fluor*. Again, it's the hardening of something which should be supple. I've had many good experiences with *Ruta* in ganglia. And again what I do these days is use castor oil externally. Castor oil rubbed in will gradually dissolve it.

Some people will get ganglia from mechanical causes. Again, it's from overuse. They've been doing some kind of physical work that involves the wrists and the hands, and that brings it on. Other people, it's more of a constitutional thing, in which case they'll need constitutional treatment as well.

Audience: Ganglion is a kind of fatty tumour, isn't it?

Ian: It's not really a fatty tumour. It's more a fibrous tumour.

Audience: So it would be like a hard (inaudible)....?

Ian: Yes. They can get really hard. Traditional allopathic treatment is to bash it with a bible. Doctors in England still recommend that. Do they do that here?

Audience: It's supposed to work.

Ian: Bible-bashing, huh?

Audience: That's what someone recommended for mine, because I developed it from twisting too many vials for too many years. He said, "Just put your hand on a table and hit it with a heavy bible. Of course there may be other problems that arise." I said, "Just forget it." It's gone down quite a lot in the past two years from not doing that.

Ian: If the body can grow these things, it can also dissolve them.

Audience: It's also referred to as "bible bump." Some people call it "bible bump." It's from bible-thumping - that brings it on.

Ian: I found, the homeopath I worked with, said the best potency for ganglia is 50M, which is pretty high, *Ruta* 50M. So I decided to try that a few times, and sure enough, if it's going to work, it works real quick. I can say that much. Whereas a 6C three times a day might do it in three months, a 50M will probably do it in ten days. That's pretty good.

Audience: (Inaudible question about fish oils and shark oil.)

Ian: As far as I know, the fish oils are usually more for internal consumption, and some of the shark oil stuff has been used as an anti-cancer agent and an immune stimulant, whereas castor oil is purely for external use. It's much more effective than things like cod liver oil and stuff. You don't want to rub those fish oils externally. Those things may be good for internal uses. And don't drink the castor oil. It's pretty toxic, unless you're really constipated, in which case, it may help.

Carpal Tunnel Syndrome

Something else I wanted to say about *Ruta*. Tendonitis, tennis elbow, anything of that kind, and also carpal tunnel syndrome - it's the number one remedy, especially, again, if you get the aetiology of overuse. If you don't have the aetiology of overuse and someone has carpal tunnel syndrome, I'll just give you some clues as to remedies. If there's been an injury, and the person has that problem, *Hypericum* or *Ruta* will usually be good. If it's very painful, shooting pains with numbness, it's more *Hypericum*.

The other main one for carpal tunnel would be *Causticum*. I mentioned that one already, especially if you get contracture developing, and especially if it's the right side. *Causticum* has a stronger affinity with the right hand, the right wrist. Remember our ex-Prime Minister Margaret Thatcher? How could you forget Mrs. Thatcher? She developed carpal tunnel syndrome, and a lot of homeopaths speculated that her remedy was *Causticum*. Who knows? She had some pretty fixed ideas! {Editor's note: I think this was a memory lapse on my part. I discussed this with colleagueas and we agreed that Lady Thatcher had suffered with Duypetren's contracture, not carpal tunnel syndrome. Still a good case for *Causticum*, I think! I.W.}

Audience: That would be with other remedies?

Ian: *Causticum*? Not necessarily. This one it could be more of a constitutional thing. It's more like the person's general tendency is towards problems in this area. And it's more likely to be chronic, more long term.

Another one I found helpful in carpal tunnel is *Guaiacum*. I mentioned that already, the one with the strange spelling, especially if you get a lot of stiffness there. I had a patient who had this problem, carpal tunnel syndrome, I think I wrote about this woman in the book. She worked in a fish and chip shop in England. So all day long, she's putting the fish and chips in and out of the oil. And that was her job all day. And she had this problem in her wrist. It was clearly from overuse, and she was due to have surgery in three days time. I just happened to go in there, and she was talking about this to a customer, and I said, "Oh, there's something that can help with that, homeopathic." She said, "Well, whatever it is, I'll try it. I'm seeing the surgeon on Thursday." I thought, "Well there's not much to lose," so I gave her *Ruta* 50M, and she was cured in twenty-four hours. She'd had the problem for three and a half months. The next day, it was gone. She was trying it to try to bring it back on again. She went to see the surgeon, and he kind of thought she had been misdiagnosed or something like that. She said, "Well, you diagnosed it!" She was pretty smart. You know, these little things. Just imagine what kind of position she's in, in terms of referrals to me. She built that whole practice for me, in the space of the next few months. And that's all I gave her.

Audience: Plus he got free fish and chips!

Ian: Free fish and chips for the rest of my life! She won't forget something like that. And she told all her customers. And she said, "Bring your cards. I want your cards on the board." She was so impressed. It's little things that we homeopaths think is poor homeopathy, treating a local problem with a first-aid remedy. To her it was the best thing. She built my whole practice.

"Ailments from playing the violin or the viola". That's what they say. I've only used *Viola-odorata* a couple of times. It also has some skin symptoms I've used it in. I don't know it that well as a remedy, but it does have an affinity with carpal tunnel and the nerves there. A strong affinity with the right wrist, so it's like *Causticum*. You found a cure on that? That's great - it has a strong affinity. Were your cases violin players?

Audience: No - from doing acupressure.

Ian: Yes. That would be a good aetiology for that kind of problem.

Audience: Would *Ruta* still be good for the other side of the wrist?

Ian: *Ruta* still has the strongest affinity that I know of. The other one that is more specific for the extensors is *Plumbum*, if you can be that specific. If the problem is the extensors, I would think of *Plumbum*. But for the flexors, *Ruta*, definitely. Housemaid's knee, tennis elbow, golfers elbow, all those kind of sports injuries. *Ruta* would be a top remedy in any sports medicine kit.

If someone has cystic lumps, I've seen this a few times, in the synovial membrane, on the joint capsule, some people get cysts there and they have surgery to get them removed, and then they regrow, and then they have scar tissue, and it's a vicious cycle. *Silica* is very, very specific for that. Someone gets cysts in the synovial membrane, give them *Silica*. I generally find that the high potency will cure that a lot faster than the low potencies. I used to try 6C daily and stuff, and it would sometimes work. And then I tried a very high potency, and it would work much faster. There's something about the very high potency, if the body is able to dissolve something quickly, it will do it very quickly on a high potency. Same with *Calc.-fluor.* Someone's got a bony spur or something, a hardening somewhere, and it's localised, a nodule in the breast, *Calc.-fluor.* really high - 50M, one dose.

Audience: The *Bellis* story! I had a indurating area in the breast. I fell against a wooden thing really hard. I thought, "I'll just see if this goes away on its own, and a month later, it hadn't. It was burning and stinging and freaking me out. I'd been lifting some stumps and gardening and straining the same day, so I took *Bellis-perennis* 30C, and in thirty seconds, it was gone. Not just felt better - it was gone.

Ian: Maybe it's your constitutional remedy? That's pretty impressive! Blows to the breast and over-exertion.

Audience: At the same time, I have an old tendon injury from a glass cut, a severed tendon, and that whole part of my hand started hurting just like it did when the tendon was cut. It hurt for hours.

Ian: There you go - a return of old symptoms. And then did it heal?

Audience: Yes. It was fine.

Ian: It brought out an old site. A good sign. You get that on a remedy, it's a good sign. I've seen that sometimes, someone has an ankle sprain, you give them *Arnica* for this, and as that heals, they come up with an old shoulder injury, or an old hip injury, within a few days. It's a good sign. They hadn't even thought to mention it. It was twenty years ago. So that remedy has gone deep.

Audience: Yes - this was an old ankle injury which turned up in the same twenty-four hours.

Ian: That usually shows that the remedy has gone deep. The person needed it for years for other things.

Audience: I had a lady. She came to me. She jammed her finger, and the pain and everything, I gave her *Hypericum* for it. She called up the next day, and she said, "I don't know whether to come over and kiss you or give you a big smack. "My finger is wonderful, but my knee is horrible" - and what was dramatic about this, this was a 30C out of my beginner's kit, and that knee had been totally nerve dead for fourteen years! She could kneel on a toy and bleed that whole area, she didn't even know. She woke up and it's completely normal. This is years down the road, and it's still normal.

Ian: That's pretty good!

Audience: Amazing! I mean it's just amazing!

Ian: I had a similar thing, someone who'd had a nerve cut, in the wrist - I think maybe they'd had carpal tunnel. This person had a nerve cut, and they had deadness in the fingers ever since and they had an injury, and they took *Hypericum* for it, and this all came back within a few days. All the sensation came back. Incredible, isn't it? But it's classic, injury to nerves, that's *Hypericum*. And yet, people are told that these things can't grow back, so we don't even think to treat them. I've had people ask me in the past, "Can nerves grow back? Can homeopathy do that?" And I've said, "No, I don't think so." But we don't know what's possible, do we? It's worth a try.

Joint Problems

I want to talk a few minutes about a few little remedies with strong joint affinities. Some of these will be more chronic joint problems, where it's not so much a first-aid situation, but it's not necessarily a constitutional problem either, where they just happen to have a chief complaint that's affecting the joints primarily. So there's a group of remedies to look at here. The first one is a relatively small remedy called *Benzoic-acid*.

It's an interesting little one. It's got a strong affinity with the kidneys and the urinary system as well as the joints. Often you'll see those two things together in the same patient. One of its best keynotes is very, very strong smelling, dark urine. Often poor elimination by the kidneys is part of the picture. It's one of the best remedies for gout. Gouty deposits. One of its best keynotes is cracking in the joints, the technical term for which is crepitation. It's when you get cracking, and you can hear it.

The other thing that I've seen *Benzoic-acid* help is bunions. Bunions, especially on the big toe. These can be very, very painful. Again, people often end up having surgery, and then they have a recurrence, and then they have more surgery. It's not a nice operation. It often takes them a long time to recovery.
Audience: Would you use high potency for that?
Ian: No, I would tend to use this in low potency, repeated. I think I only used to have it in 6X and I would give that three times a day, for a period of weeks and sometimes months. Remember it as a remedy for gout, cracking joints, especially the knees, and bunions affecting the big toe. *Lithium-carb.* is another one for cracking joints.

Anybody use that one much - *Benzoic-acid*? Anyone have any cases with it at all? It's one of those little ones that get lost so much; it's probably a polychrest, really! (Laughter.) I like the little ones.

This is a bigger one. Jane always asks the question. I always talk about *Kali-carb.* I'll take any opportunity to talk about *Kali-carb.* *Kali-carb.* is a constitutional remedy, in other words, it can affect the whole person, mentals and everything, but it's got a very, very strong affinity with the skeleton, with the whole skeletal structure, and particularly with the pelvis and the back, the sciatic nerve and the hips. So it's like the weight-bearing area of the body. Its a major remedy following pregnancy and childbirth. All kinds of structural misalignment problems, especially if they're following childbirth. Sciatica since childbirth, it would be a number one remedy. *Hypericum* would be a close competitor. Also think of it where a woman had a difficult labour, and ever since then, she's had a backache which typically will reoccur every time she has her period. So backache with the menstrual cycle, which was triggered by a difficult childbirth, usually a prolonged labour where the child got stuck, something like that.

Audience: And is the pain during the period?

Ian: It can be before, and/or during.

Audience: Ian, I had one woman who had like the symphysis pubis separated, and always felt like it never quite got back together again.

Ian: Right.

Audience: Is that more *Kali-carb*, or I was wondering if *Bellis-perennis*....

Ian: I would think of *Bellis* first. And I'd also consider *Caulophyllum*. Another thing to look for with *Kali-carb.* is a person who has lumbar back problems and what they want to do is support the back. They want to sit with a cushion in the chair so that there's something firm up against their back. Or they'll say it's O.K. if they're lying on a hard surface or a nice, firm mattress. They don't like it to be too soft. Anything that gives it too much space and flexibility will aggravate.

It's also a major remedy for hip problems, and especially the right hip. So it's got a particularly strong affinity with the right hip. If you don't know what to do, someone with right hip problems, or you've tried the constitutional, or you can't find it, I found that *Kali -carb.* has a very, very strong affinity with the right side, and it's particularly good if you've got things going from the hip down to the knee. So if you have pain which is extending from the right hip down to the right knee, that's a very strong indication for *Kali-carb*.

Audience: What kind of potency with that?

Ian: Whatever, really - 30, 200. It's one I would tend to give as a single dose, see how they respond. And repeat it, if you need to. The exception to that is someone who's got chronic arthritis, in which case I would probably start low, 6c's daily, and work your way up.

Audience: Now *Kali-carb.* is the one I remember from Kent's being the big lecture on what not to do. It scared me to death, and I had a call from another homeopath who had given it to someone who died, and she was scared she had killed him, and it was like - can you talk about that, whether there's a specific case to avoid?

Ian: Right. I think he was right in identifying it as a deep-acting remedy, which means to me that it has an affinity with deep organs and tissues. Not just tissues, but organs. So it has a deep affinity with the liver, a strong affinity with the lungs, a fairly strong affinity with the kidneys, and an affinity with the spine and with the gall bladder. I think what Kent observed was using it in things like tuberculosis, where the patient was heading deathwards anyway, and he gave a high potency usually, Kent being Kent, of a remedy that had a strong affinity with their weakest organ, and it was enough to tip them over the edge. They were headed that way anyway. It's not like the remedy killed them, but it kind of exacerbated where they were already going. I think partly due to the potency and partly because he was treating too deep, too soon. He should have probably been using organ remedies rather than constitutional remedies.

My own experience has been, outside of something like T.B., which it's unlikely that you'll get to treat much of, that you can use *Kali-carb.* like any other remedy. I've used it really a lot in arthritis, sciatica, hip-joint problems, backache, in pregnancy, during and after childbirth, and menstrual and hormonal problems and thyroid problems. It's just such a polychrest, I wouldn't hesitate to give it to someone where it's indicated. I honestly can't say I've seen it cause more aggravations or worse aggravations than any other remedy.

Audience: It made an impression on Kent.....

Ian: Yes. He probably had one bad experience with it, you know? Someone threatened to sue him after (laughter).....He got a bit scared about it. I don't know what.

It's really good if a woman's had a bad childbirth and what she's said is, "All the labour pains were in the back." If you ever hear that, even if it's years later now, she describes the pregnancy, and you say, was there anything particularly strong about the pregnancy, and she says, "Well, no, but during the labour it was all in my back. My back was killing me". If you ever hear that, *Kali-carb.* will probably be what she needs, even years later. And the chances are that woman will have on-going backache. She'll have a weak back. It's a great remedy.

Audience: Would you go for a low potency some years later from the birth?

Ian: No. If it's a clear never-well-since, I'd tend to give it higher. I only would start lower if it's a degenerative pathology, like they've got osteoarthritis or something like that. Then I would start chipping away with a 6C.

Another thing *Kali-carb.* has a lot of is oedema. A tendency to fluid retention. They have it locally. The fingers can get puffy and so on, but especially in the face, where you see that in the face, puffy around the eyes is a good little clue, the kidney weakness. What would you think of for oedema around the ankles and the feet? What would be your top remedy?

Audience: *Medorrhinum.*

Ian: Yes. *Medorrhinum* would be my number one, if you don't know what to do, and that's the chief complaint, the tendency to accumulate fluid in the ankles and the feet.

Audience: Even in a cat?

Ian: Yes, why not?

72

Sciatica

Right sided sciatica. The top remedies that I've seen effective are: *Kali-carb.*, again, *Lycopodium, Causticum* and *Chelidonium*. That group would be my top ones for right-sided sciatica. I mean, it's a big condition, sciatica, and it can often be referred to many organs. If you read Burnett's writings on sciatica, he found that sciatica was often secondary to a uterine congestion, as he called it. Or it can be from a liver weakness, and even a spleen problem. This is unheard of in allopathic diagnosis. I've certainly seen *Chelidonium* work for right-sided sciaticas, and *Chelidonium* is a liver remedy more than anything else. My suspicion was that it was sciatica secondary to a liver problem. He called it, "portal congestion," where the portal circulatory system was congested. That would produce a sciatica.

And left-sided sciatica, for your interest, *Thuja, Medorrhinum* and *Lachesis* would probably be your top group. Those are all big remedies, but they have a strong affinity with the left side. And *Rhus.-tox.* Those would be my leaders.

Audience: I had a *Rhus-tox.* failure, and *Colocynthis* did it.
Ian: In sciatica? Right or left?
Audience: Left.
Ian: Left side. Good one. Were they doubled over?
Audience: No.
Ian: What led you to *Colocynthis*?
Audience: Actually, some of the modalities.
Ian: Better pressure, or something like this?
Audience: Yes. It extended all the way down to her ankle.
Ian: Right.
Audience: They were going to do disc surgery. They were going to fuse her spine & she avoided it.
Ian: Great.
Audience: *Colocynthis*. I was amazed and happy!
Ian: It's a good remedy. And sometimes sciatica will connect to suppressed anger.
Audience: That was another indication.
Ian: Was that in the case? Right. So if you see that indication, sciatica with suppressed anger, I would think of *Colocynthis, Staphysagria* or *Causticum*. Any of those three can handle it. The more acute it is, the more it would be *Colocynthis*. People with sciatica can really, really suffer. I've seen grown men reduced to tears in a few minutes with sciatica pain. It's really, really horrible, and you know when you've found the right remedy. Instantly they get relief. And they can be

taking heavy pain killers with no relief whatsoever. If they get relief from warmth, remember *Mag.-phos.* in sciatica is very, very effective. Someone has sciatic pain and they put a hot water bottle on it and it relieves it, you can give them *Mag.-phos.* while you're working on the case and it will nearly always help. They can just take that as a pain killer. It may or may not cure. Sciatica also can be associated with worries about money, financial insecurity, in which case I would think of remedies like *Arsenicum*. If you get like a burning-type pain and you get financial anxiety with it and they're restless with it, you have an *Arsenicum* picture.

Another thing you'll see with *Kali-carb.* is they often talk about support, lacking support, needing support. It can have that in common with *Pulsatilla*.

Another little one I want to mention to you, with a strong affinity with the ankles, is *Strontium-carb.*, another one of those weird radio-active things. It's got a particularly strong affinity with sprained ankles that don't heal. So this is when you've tried everything, *Rhus*, and *Arnica* and *Ruta*, and they still have weakness, lameness or pain in an old ankle injury. *Strontium-carb.* when all else fails. They may still have some oedema or swelling or puffiness in the joint. It's very effective. Anyone used that one? It's a good one to have up your sleeve, when you've tried everything else.

Audience: Does it have an affinity with other connective tissue or other tendons in the body?

Ian: I don't know. I only know it in that context really, sprained ankles. The only other thing I know about it is that it's a remedy for post-surgical shock. Someone who goes into shock after an operation. It's also indicated for that. You'd probably have to be in the operating theatre to know that they're in it. I don't know if it's more general than that. Ankles - I think that's its main area that it homes in on.

I'm just going to mention one other for sciatica, and then we'll maybe have a little break, and that's *Valerian*. Another neglected herbal remedy, with a strong neuro-muscular affinity. And, it's got a peculiar thing, worse when a person is standing or resting on their feet, for sciatica, but better when they're walking. If you ever see that particular keynote. It's relieved as long as they're walking. If they're stood still, putting weight on the limb, it aggravates. That's *Valerian*. Another thing that it has which is peculiar is the pain in the heels. The person complains of pains in the heels. I can remember treating a guy who had pain in the heels, it was his chief complaint. And I gave him everything. I gave him absolutely everything. And I think it was ages later that I discovered this, I think he'd given up on me,

and I actually phoned him, and I said, "Would you like to try this?" Because I felt bad, taking money off him and treating him for ages and I tried all the things I could think of, and nothing helped. And he took the *Valerian.* I gave him like a 12C, it was the only thing I could find, and it instantly took it away. And he'd had this problem for years. He was so impressed. It was all he wanted anyway. I'd been trying to find all these other things to prescribe on for months.
Audience: This was in potency?
Ian: Yes. I actually gave it to him in potency, 12C, and within a day or two, it was completely gone. It was amazing.

Perceiving What is to be Cured

I saw a woman in the clinic recently. The chief complaint was problems with the extremities, fingers and hands, primarily. She had pains and numbness, and she had been given *Rhus-tox.* There were pains, numbness, stiffness. On the local symptoms, *Rhus-tox.* seemed fairly well indicated, and when she took it, she got some relief, but it didn't cure, and a different potency had pretty much the same effect. I sat in to try to get another perspective on the case.

What I noticed, first of all, this woman, I think she was seventy-one years old. And she came in and she looked a lot younger than that. She looked like someone perhaps in her fifties, so that was the first thing that struck me. The second thing was that this woman had on extremely tight jeans. So she wore quite sexy looking jeans, really, which seemed to me again unusual in a woman her age, in England, at least, maybe less so here. And she sat, and as soon as she sat, she put her hands between her legs and crossed her legs, like this. And she had a blouse on that was open to about here. So she almost fell out of this blouse. And she sat and pouted at me, whilst she was interacting with the homeopath, and between everything that she said, she would look at me and give me a pout. Not quite blow me a kiss, but it wasn't far off.

So I sat looking at this woman and thinking "there's more to this than *Rhus-tox*". There's a bigger totality here that isn't being prescribed upon.
Audience: You're almost seeing the bigger totality.
Ian: Yes. It's true. I mention this to emphasise the idea of perceiving what has to be cured. We don't always see it even when it smacks us in the face. We get too focused on the chief complaint, or whatever is bothering the person, and we don't always see that there's a

much bigger picture sitting just behind that, which is actually more characteristic, more indicative of the remedy. Now what remedy would come to mind?

Audience: *Sepia, Hyos., Platina, Anacardium.*

Ian: Why *Anacardium*?

Audience: She exposes herself.

Ian: Right. She was a sexy woman. That's really what came across. I personally wouldn't associate that with *Anacardium* that strongly. She oozed sexuality. The two that we looked at strongly were *Hyosyamus* and *Platina*. There was something that was so overtly sexual, that all her energy seemed to be there, rather than in the fingers. When we looked up *Platina*, it had all of the symptoms that she described in the fingers. It had the typical numbness and the pains just as she described it. So we gave her *Platina*. Then the other day, Pam had a case here......

Pam: Oh, it was totally casual. I was taking down some things, just during a chat. I said, "Tell me a few things, and I'll see if there's anything I can toss at you...."

Ian: So the similarities were that this is someone who appears to have a local problem from a first-aid situation. She dropped something on her foot several years ago, and she's had problems ever since. So she has tingling, numbness, swelling and finds it hard to wear her shoes. She has a diagnosis which I liked, "Reflexive neurological vascular dystrophy." That's pretty good, isn't it?

Audience: Sounds reimbursable.

Ian: This is where it's at, isn't it? So it's right-sided, she gets tingling in her right hand, worse at night, sometimes burning, sometimes aching. She's got a history of both ovarian and uterine cancer, and she has irregular menses which are very light, with pains in the left ovary, and the thing Pam has written on the bottom of her notes, with emphasis, is "high sex drive." Which is something that you know about from knowing her elsewhere?

Pam: Yes - she talks about sex all of the time.

Ian: So again, it's a question of where is the person's energy tied up? This is what we always have to try to keep a perspective on. My guess is that this lady would also need *Platina*.

Now sometimes what appears to be a local problem is more of a general picture. It goes back to the discussion we had earlier. And sometimes it's the other way around. Sometimes we focus too general, we're looking for that general remedy that covers everything when what the person actually needs is a local remedy, because they've never been well since a local trauma, or something of that kind. And I try not to know which it might be when I'm taking a case.

I try to have no opinion about where it might be coming from, and really let the person speak energetically as well as with their mouth. Just let them speak to you. It doesn't really matter. The main thing is just to start somewhere. You start the treatment based on where you think it is.

One of the things I learned from Clarke, I think he was probably one of the most skilled at this, and he used a nice analogy to describe it. He said, "Sometimes, in homeopathy, we need a microscope, we need to focus right down. And sometimes you need a telescope. You need to see the big picture from a long distance." Try to keep that in mind. We don't know. It depends on what you're looking at whether the microscope is the best tool, or whether a telescope is the best tool. And as homeopaths we need both, and I would say equally.

In a lot of the cases I've supervised, the problem has been that the homeopath is looking too general, too broad, more times, I'd say, than the other way around. So most of us who are trained to prescribe constitutionally, we habitually go for the bigger picture. We're just trained to do that, and we miss the fact that this person has never been well since a bang on the head or since an injection, or something quite local, or something which is superimposed on the big picture. It might have been a grief or a humiliation or something of that kind. And actually what they need is a remedy for that first, and then a general remedy, maybe afterwards.

So if you treat someone, and your experience is that what you thought was the problem, and you're aiming your remedy at that, what it tends to do is produce a palliation. In other words, as long as they take the remedy they feel better. You stop the remedy, it comes back. That's one response to look out for. That should be a little red flag. It's not a bad thing, but it's telling you something about the level on which you're prescribing. So palliation is one possibility.

The second thing to look out for is new things emerging, new problems emerging quickly after the person gets relief of the local problem. So you treat the knee, and the knee's fine, and now they've got shoulder pain, and you treat the shoulder and it's fine, and now the neck hurts. And you treat that, and now they've got a headache, so it seems like you're chasing it around. That's the second scenario.

And the third is that the local problem gets better, but there's a general aggravation. They say that my energy's gone down, or my sleep has become disturbed, or my menstrual cycle has gone off since

I took that remedy, something of this kind. That's relatively unusual, but it will happen occasionally. The local remedy will do something, but it's not really curative. It's just changed the picture in some way.

Any of these responses all say that there's a bigger totality that needs looking at. So whenever you get any of those: palliation, new problems emerging, and they have to be new, it's not a return of old symptoms, it's something they didn't have before, or there's a general demise. If any of those happen, what you have to do is put away the microscope and take out the telescope. What you need is a bigger picture, a broader perspective.

If, on the other hand - I know that this is kind of obvious to many of you, but I want to remind you of it anyway, if on the other hand you get the response that the person in themself is better, but the chief complaint gets worse and stays worse. It's not just that they've had a temporary aggravation, but it becomes worse and stays there, it's worse than before they consulted you, it's not just temporarily aggravated in the process of cure. They come back a few weeks later and their arthritis is bothering them more now than it was before they consulted you. And it's got new modalities, especially. Look out for that. The chief complaint has new symptoms or new modalities.

So in other words, when you took the case, there wasn't much to go on in terms of the joints, so you prescribed generally, and now they come back, and they say, "These joints are burning, they're waking me at three in the morning", and it's gotten real specific, whereas before, it was vague. If any of these happen, what the person is telling you is that you need to go from the general to the particular. You need to swap the telescope for the microscope. The local problem is calling out - "it's me that needs the remedy now".

And maybe you weren't able to see that at the first visit, and that is totally O.K. Sometimes it will only reveal itself in the process of the treatment. You know, when you first take the case, quite often the local modalities are not quite crisp enough to determine the remedy, and it's only in the process of the treatment that it becomes more a picture in itself. You know the totality in homeopathy is only three symptoms, really. That's what Hering said, the three-legged stool. We have the idea that the totality means everything. It means three characteristics: the location, a good modality, aetiology, concomitant, whatever.

So the two cases I've just described - what was needed was the bigger picture, whereas what was presenting was a local problem. The chances are the local remedy wouldn't cure either of these two women, because there's a bigger picture presenting. The confirmation, usually, is that when you see the bigger picture remedy, you'll usually find that the local problem is embraced by it, it's encompassed within it, so the same remedy covers both. Whenever you find that, it's usually a good prognosis.

Cases & Further Questions

Does anyone have cases or people that you've thought about treating, or might consider treating, that you want to ask about and that are relevant to today?

Audience: This is somebody I've been working with for a while that I keep helping a little bit, but not very much. What's coming up now, well she's had high blood pressure going on for a long time, but she's developed a pterygium, a little lump on the eye, and she said her eye was feeling sore, as if somebody had hit her, and it was getting bloodshot, and I gave her *Cocculus*, and it went away and it came back, and then I gave her *Calcarea* and it went away and came back a couple of weeks later. One question I have is about whether - this is somebody who no way at all could I see her as a constitutional *Calcarea*, but it covers the pterygium which is a pretty small rubric, it has a high blood pressure picture that does seem to fit her, and it has the connection with overwork. So where you have the situation where a whole bunch of stuff seems to fit, and yet it seems to really not fit in a fundamental way, is that a go or a no go? That's one question.
Ian: The bottom line is we can only judge by results, and if your experience is in treating that what you're doing isn't curing. . .
Audience: Well, the other thing that happened, okay, so she had one dose and then a day or so ago, she said it was coming back, so I told her to take it again, so I don't really know what's going to happen.
Ian: Right.
Audience: I also never know like the whole issue of how often to re-dose, I get confused, because on the one hand, my own prescriber, if a 200 doesn't last at least six months, he says, "That's it, it's the wrong remedy," but other people - I know it has something to do with the situation, but I really feel confused about how to gauge it. She's under a tremendous amount of ongoing stress, so I don't know if that justifies it being used up.
Ian: Well, certainly the life situation that the person's in will to a large

extent determine how long they'll benefit from a curative remedy, as will the intensity of the disease process. Like we talked about earlier, if someone's got a high fever or something that's quite intense, they'll use up the energy of the remedy very quickly, so they'll need frequent repetition. However, if the remedy is similar enough to alleviate, but not similar enough to cure, you will also see that they use it up quickly. It's palliative rather than curative. People will need more and more of it to get the same benefit. Any of those is possible.

The only way you'll find out if it's curative or not is to give it again. What's happening is, there's a point at which you'll know, because palliation will turn into cure if the intervals between doses get longer. Then you know that it's a curative remedy. If those intervals get shorter, then you know it is only ever going to be a palliative remedy. The only way you find that out is by repeating it. Whenever she says, "I was better for a week, but now it's come back", so you give another dose. If she then says, "I was better for three days and now it's come back," the chances are it's not a curative remedy.

Audience: No, it's a couple weeks. So then do you have an impression? My understanding of *Calc.-carb.* as a constitutional remedy is a person with a solid build and a phlegmatic disposition, and that whole thing, and she's not like that at all. And yet, for a certain picture, it fits real well.

Ian: Isn't homeopathy wonderful? You see, the beauty and the curse of homeopathy is that it's so subjective. We prescribe according to what we see. So the prescription is as much a reflection of the prescriber as of the patient, and it's often the case that a patient going to three different homeopaths will get three different well-indicated remedies. Who's to say that they wouldn't all help? I really don't subscribe to the, "There's only one remedy that will help" idea. That seems ridiculous to me. I don't think that there's only one therapy that will help either.

However, let me give you a tip for this person, and that is, there's one remedy that I know will help this person with both of her health problems. And that remedy is sunlight. How does she get on with the sun?

Audience: She likes it. She doesn't have much chance to get out. She does try to get out. I passed that along to her about blood pressure after your last lecture.

Ian: Both of these conditions can be induced by sunlight deprivation. Both of them. I don't know if you were here when I talked about a famous case of a whole group of native people who developed pterygium in all the males, and it was after it became trendy to wear sunglasses. So they were no longer getting the sunlight in their eyes, and because of that, they all developed pterygium. I told that story in London, and there was a woman who sat in the front row of the seats, and she said, "I've got pterygium." And I asked her, "When did it come on?" And she said, "I used to live in South Africa, and it came on when I moved to England. When I moved to England, my eyesight went funny. I started wearing glasses. Not only did she move away from the sun, but she also put glasses on full-time. For the first time, she developed pterygium. She said, "I can't take the light now. I'm photophobic."

So we have to get the sunlight in the eyes. It's clinically proven that sunlight in the eyes will lower the blood pressure and it will certainly alleviate and in many cases cure this condition.
Audience: But that needs to be on the order of hours per day, doesn't it?
Ian: No, it doesn't.
Audience: How long?
Ian: Something like half an hour a day, if it's regular, and as long as the eyes are unshaded. That would be sufficient. The regular repetition is better than one long occasional exposure - one day a week is not as good as half an hour a day, every day. So you could do that while you're figuring out the case.

Another thing you might think about is that these are what you might call *solar conditions*. In the alchemy tradition, every organ in the body is ruled by one of the outer planets. They include the sun as one of the planets. And the sun rules both the heart and the blood and the eyes. So this woman has a solar condition. She's got sun diseases.
Audience: As opposed to a mars condition?
Ian: Yes. It's not mars, it's not venus, this is sun, these are sun diseases, both of the things that she complains of. So I would be looking for a remedy that has a solar affinity.
Audience: Does Boericke mention those?
Ian: *Aurum* would be one..........
Audience: I tried *Aurum*....
Ian: So you look at gold, affinity with the heart; *Lachesis* - affinity with the heart; *Sulphur* - heart and circulation. What I would do would be to look in the rubrics that you're looking at, and see which of these remedies has got a solar affinity. *Belladonna, Glonoine, Lachesis, Sulphur, Aurum* - the *Aurums* in general, all the golds have this, and salt, of course, as a remedy.
Audience: Robin Murphy tells what planets rule the remedies in his

Materia Medica - do you have that?

Ian: Yes, if you look in Murphy's *Materia Medica*, it has a chapter, or a section in the back. So you can look at sun, and you get a whole group of remedies there. Every remedy under the sun! So I would check that out. It might just give you an insight into the case. I just had a quick look at the pterygium section, and the ones that would be solar remedies there would be: *Euphrasia, Lachesis* and *Sulphur* - they would be the strongest. And look at *Belladonna*. O.K.? It's something to think about. Anyone else got cases?

Audience: Scoliosis.

Ian: Scoliosis of the spine?

Audience: Yes.

Ian: We can talk about that. In fact I think I've even got some notes on it. The main remedy that I know of is *Calc.-phos*. Let's see if we've got anything else here. Yes, we could touch on that. All of the *Calcium* salts, in terms of constitutionals, can have a tendency to this. Scoliosis of the spine. So you've got *Calc.-carb., Calc.-fluor, Calc. -phos., Calc.-sulph.* and even *Calc.-iod*. So depending on what was together with it, you could look at those as a group. The other main ones would be *Phosphorus*, if it's more of a tubercular type, you'd look at *Phosphorus* and *Calc.-phos*. When I've seen that, especially in children, they've been very tubercular. And also *Silica*. Those are the main ones that I know of.

Audience: Do you ever use *Syphilinum* or something like that?

Ian: Yes, depending on what's there in their history. On that alone, I wouldn't. But yes if there's a family history or a medical history that supports it. If you don't know what to do, I would look at *Calc.-phos.*, and *Calc-fluor*. You could do those as tissue salts, while you're working on the case. It would probably improve things. The person may also benefit from bodywork of some kind, energy bodywork in preference to manipulation.

Audience: Do you think of the tissue salts as good tonics?

Ian: Well, they're more than that. They're curatives as well. They're curative remedies for many, many people. I think a lot of people are sick not just energetically. They also have deficiency diseases. Some people get around that with using vitamins and minerals and supplementation. I don't use that extensively, but some practitioners do. My substitution for that is to use tissue salts a lot. I think you can do a lot that vitamins and minerals would do by using tissue salts, because you're improving their absorption, plus you're also feeding the body with some of the basic salts. There's not a whole lot, but they're amongst the most important ones.

Audience: Have you had any experience with whiplash?

Ian: Yes. This is a good area. This is an area where you could have a whiplash clinic, and you could really demonstrate homeopathy's effectiveness. We have several remedies for that. Number one of course is *Hypericum*. If you see someone who has just had a whiplash, or they've never been well since a whiplash injury, I would try *Hypericum* first before anything else. And I generally would start off with a single dose first, relatively high potency for that, like a 200c and upwards. If you see someone where the *Hypericum* doesn't help or it only partially helps, and especially if it's long term, you know, they did it a long time ago, and they've never been well since, the second best remedy I've found is *Nat.-sulph*. I can't even remember where I came across that.

Audience: Because of headaches afterward?

Ian: Yes. Headaches after head injury, and things like that.

Audience: And also epilepsy after head injury?

Ian: Possibly. It's got an affinity with the whole cerebro-spinal fluid mechanism.

Audience: Are there other whiplash remedies?

Ian: There's a couple others I want to mention. Sometimes whiplash will develop into other things, like a torticollis I've seen, where a person gets stuck to one side, the head drawn to one side, because they've been in a lot of pain, and then they start tightening up, so it develops into other problems. It kind of goes into other areas. The torticollis group of remedies is a group in itself. *Rhus-tox.* is one of the strongest. Look for the stiffness. If the main thing that remains is the stiffness, *Rhus-tox.* is what they need. Another one of the strongest ones for torticollis is *Causticum*. Again, you get that stiffness, contraction, rigidity, tightening up. I've also seen *Ignatia* be very good, post-whiplash, where you get spasms. This is where it comes and goes. They think it's better, and then, especially if they're under stress, suddenly it goes again and they feel the neck pain come on. So if you ever see that intermittent spasm, post whiplash, it's usually *Ignatia*. *Ignatia* is often a good one for ailments from injury to the back of any kind. Someone's been in a car accident and they've got a spinal injury and they've had problems ever since. You try *Hypericum* and it doesn't work, have a look at *Ignatia*. And often it's just the muscles going into spasm, and then they pull the spine out and cause other problems.

If you get someone and they have torticollis and it's drawn to the left, like this, so the head starts getting pulled to the left, the two strongest remedies there are *Lycopodium* and *Phosphorus*, where the drawing is to the left side. And if it's more to the right, *Causticum* is probably the top one, and there's another small remedy, which is very specific for this, called *Lachnanthes*. It's the only place I've ever used it, torticollis drawn to the right, *Lachnanthes*. I've seen that work. And *Lycopodium* again. *Lycopodium* can be either side, right or left. Those are the ones I've seen help most.

Also, don't forget *Arnica*. If someone has whiplash, generally speaking, they've been in an accident, they've also had shock, they've probably had bruising elsewhere. Sometimes, the only reason it's not clearing up is that they didn't get *Arnica* when they needed it. High potency *Arnica* is always worth a shot. *Hypericum* and *Nat.-sulph.* would be the top two. *Ignatia* and *Rhus-tox.* coming in after those.

Audience: And a tendency to head injury? And sadness after head injury, depression?

Ian: Mental changes.........talking of which, that was another case when I sat in on a clinic, another guy came in and his chief complaint was catarrh, sinus catarrh, mucus, catarrh in his throat, so he was constantly hawking and coughing up, and it's thick, yellow-green, and it's especially bad between 4:00 and 5:00 in the morning. So I had a quick look in the repertory, and the main one that came out was *Nat.-sulph.* It had the type of phlegm that he had and it had the time aggravation that he had, and I looked at this guy. Once I saw *Nat.-sulph.* in there, I looked at him, and I thought, "This guy is a depressive." He's carrying something quite heavy that he's not talking about. This is the beauty of knowing remedies and being able to ask leading questions. If you get a hint of the remedy from the physicals, you can then ask a question based on your knowledge of that remedy, and see what else is there. I just asked him, straight away, as a confirmation, I said, "Do you ever get down and depressed?" And the guy has tears in his eyes instantly, as soon as I asked the question. And I said, "Can you just say something about that?" And it turned out that it was since he had become estranged from his wife - they had separated acrimoniously, and she had taken the children - and he wasn't allowed to see them. If you look in the rubric, *"Estranged from family,"* *Nat.-sulph.* is the main remedy. So it was like a general remedy for him. It was quite a confident prescription. And I could see, just from how he responded to my question, that he was suicidal, or had been, and I asked the person who was his homeopath later, and he said, "Oh, yeah, he had already mentioned that at an earlier visit, that he had suicidal tendencies." There is no substitute for knowing materia medica.

I sat in with a guy for a number of months. He was one of the best clinicians I ever saw, and his gift was, people would come in and they would talk keynotes to him. It was like they had been reading Boericke in the waiting room. They would just sit there and tell him keynotes, and he would look at me and say, "What's the remedy?" And while I was with him, I knew the remedy every time! I felt totally invincible. And when I was in my own practice, it took hours, and no one ever told me keynotes, and so I studied what he did. One of the things I learned was that he was a master of materia medica. He knew it inside out. And so once he got a few hints from the patient, he would be down to a couple of remedies, and then he would immediately fire back a couple of questions, you know, just bounce them off the person. "You like salt, do you?" He'd just look them right in the eye and say, "You like salt, don't you?" And they would tell him if they did or they didn't. But nine times out of ten, it was just spot on. They would go, "Wow, how did you know? I *crave* salt." They would come back with a positive response, nearly always, and that was it, that ended his case taking. He'd say, "Thanks." He would just grin. They would tell him two things, and he would ask one thing to confirm it, and he would stop taking the case. Ten or twelve minutes.

Audience: Is this the guy who saw a huge number of patients?

Ian: Yes - he used to see between thirty and thirty-five patients a day, four and a half days a week. When I saw him, he'd been doing it for about thirty-three years. You could say he'd had a bit of experience! And it really showed. People just came in, sat down, and they just spilled the beans. His knowledge of materia medica was superb, second to none. And really, he only used Boericke. I never saw him use a repertory once. I asked him about that and he said, "Repertory, yeah, I've got one somewhere. It's in one of those cabinets."

Audience: Do you think that people know if they've got a two-hour appointment with you, and if they only have twenty minutes, it's going to change how they reveal themselves to you?

Ian: Absolutely. That was one of his keys. I asked him about that, and he said, "Absolutely right." He'd tried many approaches to practice. He used to have long appointments and stuff. He said, "If you give 'em an hour, they'll take an hour. "

Audience: I mean, it's a rule for everything else in life. I don't know why it wouldn't fit this.

Ian: Exactly. People will expand to fill the available space. And every homeopath knows that they give you the clincher on the way out. Right? So many times they give you the best information when they walk out the door, so the sooner you get them to that point, the better! And that was his strategy. The other thing he used to do, he never used to put the heating on, so it was always freezing in his clinic. I'd say, "Could we have some heat in here?" He'd just look at me, and he said, "Make them too comfortable and they'll want to stay too long." He was a bit mean. He had a bit of an edge to him, but he was a lot of fun.

Audience: You would get a modality that way. The ones that were worse cold.....

Ian: Exactly. They'd either come in and complain, or they wouldn't. They'd take something off. He was a superb observer. That was the other thing he had. He was observing people the moment they came into the waiting room. He'd nip out in the waiting room and have a peep from the pharmacy. And often he'd have the remedy just on that, before they even came in. He'd kind of nudge me and say, "Watch this. *Pulsatilla.*" Before they even said anything. The patient would come in and burst into tears, and he'd just sit there with a big grin. He'd do it over and over and over again. I think more than anything else, what I learned from him was that materia medica is where it's at. Homeopathy *is* materia medica. It's knowing the remedies, and being flexible enough to give what you see, and being *prepared* to give what you see. That's what he did routinely. He'd never talk himself out of a remedy, which I used to do, and most people I know have done, often. As soon as he saw the remedy, he'd give it. And he wouldn't ask any more questions. He said, "If I ask any more questions at this point, I'll get confused." So he knew that, and he was willing to trust that. And he had such good rapport skills that he knew that people would come back anyway, whether they got better or not. They enjoyed being in his presence. So of course they came back. They came back to have a nice chat with him, because he was a great guy. And they had faith in him, because he had such strong faith in his remedies and that homeopathy would help them. He just enthused people to get well. There's a lot to be said for that. People felt better just being in his aura. I could sit with him a whole day. I'd lost count, we were at number twenty-six or something, they were just in and out, in and out, and at the end of the day, he was still buzzing. He wasn't drained. I was like, "Oh my God." He was amazing, just amazing.

And he was the first homeopath that I really saw demonstrate clinical prescribing, giving people what they want. "What's your problem?" He'd give them a remedy for it. "You've got migraines?" He'd give them a migraine remedy. And then he'd ask them about their kids. "How's your children? Oh, having trouble at school? Here, give them this. How's your husband? Oh, he snores, does he? Give him a dose of this." He'd send them out with a whole pack. And I learned

86

that from him. He was never hesitant to give it away. You know, he wasn't thinking, "I'm not getting paid for this one." He just gave it away, gave it away, gave it away. Give this one to your dog, this one to your cat, this one to your husband. Everybody went out with a pack of remedies. All the families were treated and stuff. Half the people he never even saw. He had the busiest practice of anyone I've ever known in England. It doesn't come from keeping it all tight and closed and all that stuff. His success came from giving it away, really freely, I think. That is what he did. But he loved it, too. I've worked with other people in homeopathy, and I wondered why they were doing it. Their experience was, "This is hard work, it's drudgery." You know, they didn't enjoy reading the remedies. They'd get depressed whenever they opened the repertory. All this kind of thing.

Audience: Everybody in school!

Ian: It really makes you wonder, doesn't it?

Audience: Yes, but they'll feel better soon.

Ian: Well, he never went to school. I think that was one of his advantages. He did a correspondence course or something. And he learned some things off a doctor who was quite good. And then he just set up shop. He thought, "I can do this," and off he went.

Osteoporosis

Audience: Could you talk about osteoporosis?

Ian: Yes. That was also on my list. You're filling in the blanks for me very nicely. Okay, let's have a look at some osteoporosis remedies. Brittle bones. I just read something in England, a couple of weeks ago. They estimate that one third of women in their fifties now in England, over the age of fifty-five or something, are now on hormone replacement therapy, supposedly to prevent osteoporosis. I'm sure it's not that different here. A lot of women have been pushed onto H.R.T. to prevent osteoporosis, despite the fact that it increases the risk of various types of cancer and other things which they probably omit to mention, breast cancer primarily. There's a strong correlation.

A couple of things about osteoporosis generally, first of all. One is, an excessive protein diet will increase a predisposition to osteoporosis many, many fold. So excess meat consumption is one of the leading contributory factors. The incidence in vegetarian women is very, very low, by comparison, along with many other diseases, by the way, but that is one where the relationship is very strong. One of the things that's been demonstrated with that, the high protein diet, it seems to increase the load on the kidneys. One of the side effects of that is that calcium gets leeched out by the kidneys. So less meat consumption is one thing. The second thing is that weight bearing exercise is important in the treatment plan and particularly yoga, tai chi or chi kung are the most powerful things. There's a study done, I think it was done in China, where they tested different techniques including allopathy, Chinese medicine, and they also did chi kung on osteoporosis and other bone diseases of the lower limbs and hips, and way, way above anything, including the Chinese medicine, were the chi kung exercises in terms of its effectiveness. It had a much higher cure rate, and it had the best rate for long term prevention. Some therapies could relieve it, but didn't stop it from coming back. The only thing that stopped it from coming back in the majority was chi kung. And what does chi kung involve? For the most part, it involves standing still, doing nothing. Most chi kung exercises are just standing, in a relaxed posture, with the knees bent. And the classic exercise is the 'stand like a tree'. That's all you have to do. And it's so simple, who would do it? It's too ridiculous. "Give me drugs, give me hormones any day, but don't make me stand like a tree!" It's been clinically proven, if you can get a woman with osteoporosis to stand like a tree for five or ten minutes, or as long as she can comfortably stand, and gradually build up to ten minutes or so every morning, every night. If someone does that for a period of weeks or months, x-rays will prove that she'll actually start to reverse osteoporosis, with no other changes in diet or medicine or regimen, that alone will do it. So if you can get your patients doing that, they'll do very well. Of course, what they really want is some pills.

The other thing I'll remind you of is sunlight. If someone doesn't get regular sunlight exposure, their ability to metabolise calcium efficiently will be diminished. Regular sunlight or ultraviolet light has to go into the eyes on a regular basis, and it has to hit the retina unfiltered by spectacles, contact lenses, glass, or anything else. And most of us spend ninety-odd percent of the day indoors, or behind glass, or wearing spectacles, so this is a kind of cultural obstacle to cure. The other condition that can be helped a lot by that is osteoarthritis. Osteoporosis and osteoarthritis both benefit from regular sunlight exposure. If the person says they can't stand the sun or they can't get out, then they should use ultraviolet or a full spectrum lamp, which you can buy, and just bathe the eyes in that, half an hour a day.

Audience: For people who wear glasses, there used to be one or two companies that made full-spectrum lenses, but they don't any more. There's no way to get full spectrum glasses.

Ian: Right. You have to throw them away for half an hour a day.

It's hard, I know! The other thing that sunlight will improve is your eyesight. The sun rules the eyes. You can also strengthen the eyesight with regular sunlight, or ultraviolet light exposure. There are so many conditions which are clinically proven to benefit from this. . .

Audience: You can go out and do your chi kung stand like a tree in the sun.

Ian: Exactly. Stand like a tree in the sunlight.

Audience: Now you won't have to think about walking into anything.....

Ian: Exactly. It's completely non-hazardous, non-toxic, and it's free.

Audience: And on that note, I'm going outside.

Ian: Don't forget to take your lenses out!

So that's like the generals, and then there are the remedies, which is what you're really interested in, right? The main remedy for osteoporosis is *Calc.-phos.* So you want to feed those tissues with a form of calcium that the body can utilise. Regular calcium supplementation does not work for osteoporosis. It's giving the body calcium in a way that it cannot use.

Audience: Would it be fine to do that while someone is taking *Calc. -fluor.* as a tissue salt too?

Ian: Oh yes. You can mix two or three of them together very happily. *Calc.-phos.* is number one. *Calc.-fluor.* will also help osteoporosis. So sometimes I've used a combination which, I think you can buy it ready mixed, certainly in England. What it contains is *Calc.-phos., Calc.-fluor.,* and *Silica,* and it's for the bones, hair, teeth and connective tissue. So it's marketed as a combination tissue salt. They're all in a 6X potency. Or you could mix it up yourself, I'm sure. That would be an ideal combination for osteoporosis: feeding those tissues, standing like a tree, looking at the sun, then you do the constitutional remedy. Constitutional treatment alone will not cure that condition, because it's part nutritional, part hormonal, part environmental, part diet, so I think it's more appropriate to look for a programme of things.

Audience: Do you do that then twice a day, three times a day?

Ian: The tissue salts I would say three times a day, generally. And I've had people on them for months with no ill effect. The body seems to utilise them very well. The constitutionals you'll be looking at will often be one of the *Calcium* salts, *Calc.-carb.* or *Calc.-phos.* will often be the underlying constitutional. They have a weakness there or a tendency, or it could be a *Phosphorus* or *Silica* type. So any of those general remedies with a bone affinity could be the constitutional type.

Osgood-Schlatter's Disease

Another disease - I don't know if you see much of it here, but the same remedies come up - is Osgood-Schlatters. Do you see that here? Osgood-Schlatters disease. It sounds pretty fancy, but it's not really. What is it?

Audience: It's bone growth in the legs that is growing too rapidly in children.

Ian: Yes. It's a variation on growing pains, essentially. Your number one remedy is *Calc.-phos.*, and number two is probably *Silica*. And also look at *Phosphorus*. And most kids who have this will need *Tuberculinum*.

Audience: You see this a lot - I've seen it a lot in adults. They have pains resulting from that.

Ian: You mean, since this? They had this as a child, and now they have ongoing bone and joint problems. Is that the kind of thing you're describing?

Audience: Yes, or it would be more of an example where it's constitutionally treated. I've seen a lot of like chiropractic students with it. I've seen a lot of adults who have that.

Ian: Right. I've not seen it so much in adults. Or if I have, it's diagnosed as something else, osteoarthritis or something like that. But it's the same group. You're looking at your remedies with strong bone affinities. In children, from what I've seen, they've nearly always been tubercular type kids. If you don't know what else to do, give them *Calc.-phos.* I've given *Calc.-phos.* many times without even having seen the child and it just cures it, just as a tissue salt. That one, any paediatrician should know that. To me that's professional negligence, the fact that they don't know about *Calc.-phos.* for this. It's negligence, because it works so consistently and so simply, with no side-effects. It's ridiculous that they don't know about it. I just give it away to anybody, any opportunity I get.

Bone Cancer

Audience: You mentioned bone cancer also.

Ian: Yes. I could just touch on that a little bit, some remedies in bone cancer. Bone cancer is most often secondary to a cancer elsewhere, which may or may not have been "cured." You know, often a woman has breast cancer, and when the breast has been removed, it's supposedly cured and now one day, she's got bone cancer, and it's treated as a new disease. Sometimes it will pop up as an osteoma, as a primary. In some cases you'll see it as a primary, and in other cases it's a secondary.

One of the things with bone cancer is that the person is invariably in a lot of pain, and that is mostly what the person's complaining of. You have to keep in mind that the remedy has to cover that, and so the ideal that you're looking for is a remedy that covers the pain and that has an affinity with the cancerous process. That's the way I try to narrow it down. So, if the remedy only covers the pain, an example there would be *Eupatorium-perf.*, it could give very effective pain relief, but it doesn't have an affinity with the disease process, so the chances are that it's not going to do anything curative. It's not going to help to halt the progress of the disease at all. They'll just get relief, but that relief can be very valuable and it can help buy you some time, and it can help keep the patient off of morphine and drugs. I don't say that to underestimate the value of it. What I say is keep in mind the limitations. This would be the stop point of *Eupatorium*. It would give great pain relief, but with no real curative effect, low or high potency, whatever you give. It's not going to cure the underlying cancer. It just doesn't have that kind of affinity. Whereas, if you look at remedies such as *Phosphorus* and *Symphytum*, and the *Aurum* salts, and also *Hekla-lava*, taken from the volcanic mountain in Iceland, these ones all have an affinity with the bone and with the cancerous process.

Audience: Is there a rubric for the cancerous process?

Ian: Do you have Robin Murphy's *Repertory*? That's where I recommend you look. You can look in generals or in bones. In generals, you'll find a whole section on the different types of cancer, and if you look in the bone section, you'll find *cancer of the bones* on page 198 in the new edition. He has two *Aurums* in there: *Aurum -iodatum* and *Aurum-muriaticum*. He also has *Cadmium-muriaticum*. The *Cadmiums* are very, very useful remedies for people with all types of cancer. And *Cadmium-sulph.* is particularly good for people on chemotherapy. If someone's undergoing chemotherapy and you don't know what to do, at least you can give them *Cadmium-sulph.* while you're figuring it out. I generally use a 30c and they take it as needed. It will help minimise the side-effects of chemotherapy very effectively, and it also helps keep their energy up. He also has *Conium* in there, and the same ones I've just mentioned, *Hekla-lava, Phosphorus,* and *Symphytum. Symphytum* is Comfrey, remember, also known as Knitbone. This one you can use as an herbal tincture together with whatever remedy you see is indicated. So if you think that the patient needs *Phosphorus*, I would put them on potentized *Phosphorus* plus Comfrey tincture. *Symphytum* as an herbal tincture, and have them take that, five drops, three times a day, in some water, in addition to the potentized remedy. There is no time for giving one remedy and waiting six months. It's inappropriopathy in a case like that. You need to err on the side of treating much more aggressively and more responsively to what's going on, and do several things at once. There should be a diet and a detox., a herbal tincture, a potentized remedy, anything really that you think will help to promote health.

I remember a while ago someone asking me, she said she worked in a hospital, and someone she knew in the hospital was really suffering a lot with bone cancer, and was there a remedy that could help her? I said, "Yeah, yeah, what's the symptoms?" She said, "Really, I don't know, that's the trouble, I can't take her case, she's under the doctor and I'm just working there as a nurse, and so on." I said, "Well, you've seen her." She said, "Yeah, I go in and dress her every day and this kind of thing." I said, "What's your observation?" She said, "This woman is just desperate, she's desperate, and she's on a lot of drugs." I said, "What does she say?" And she said, "She hasn't told me anything about the case." I said, "What *has* she told you?" You have to work on the assumption that patients will tell you one way or another what they need. She said, "At night, when I go in and turn her or give her a medication, all she keeps saying is, "If I don't get some relief from this pain, I'd rather not be here." "If I don't get some relief, this is so bad, I'd rather die than endure this." I said, "Okay, what remedy do you know that has an affinity with the bones that would like to die?" This is *Aurum*. So she went back and got some *Aurum* 6's and asked the woman if she'd like to try it, and she said, "Yes, I'll try anything." She started taking *Aurum* 6c, three or four times a day. Within a few days, she's off the drugs, and she's completely pain free, just on the *Aurum*, just taking it as needed. In her case, it didn't cure the disease. She died a few weeks later, but she was pain-free and drug-free. So that was still a great benefit to the patient. And she was completely lucid. She wasn't drugged up, and very grateful.

I have the assumption there's always something you can do, even if I haven't seen the patient, even if *they* haven't seen the patient. If you just stay open, and use what you're given, usually you can try something, and you still have got a fair chance of getting some relief.

Arthritis & Sacro-iliac Joint Problems

Audience: Any suggestions for arthritis? Or problems with the sacroiliac joint?

Ian: Arthritis - that's a biggie. The sacroiliac joint - I wanted to mention that before we go. *Calc. -phos.* again, surprisingly, is a very, very commonly needed remedy in those things. That combination, *Calc.-phos.* and *Calc.-fluor.*, will do a lot for sacroiliac joints, especially if they keep going out. Include the *Calc.-fluor.* Some people keep repeatedly having problems in that area. Another main remedy that is very good for relieving that is *Aesculus*, which is the horse chestnut. *Aesculus* has got a very strong affinity with the sacroiliac region, and also the lumbo-sacral area of the back. And very severe pains. A person often describes it as they feel as if the back's been broken. Severe stuff.

Another one that has similar pains - it might surprise you - is *Antimonium-tart.* Most of you will know that one as a remedy for lungs, respiratory problems, chest, coughs, and so on, but it also has a really strong affinity with the sacroiliac and the lumbo-sacral region, and it has one of the worst backaches you can imagine. It feels like the back is broken. And if you see someone with a really terrific lumbar back pain, and they're in so much pain they're in a sweat, they're breaking out in a sweat, in agonies, *Antimonium-tart.* 200 will often relieve that like a charm. I learned that from Clarke. It was in Clarke's *Prescriber*, one of those little things, you read it and you file it away somewhere, and then one day you see a case. Those are the main ones I know for the sacroiliac.

Audience: Do you know any more sacroiliac joint remedies that may be related with females and reproductive organs, where there's a crossover?

Ian: Yes. There is one that has that strongly, and that would be *Cimicifuga*. It has a strong affinity and it's also a uterine remedy. This is the one that has two names. Sometimes it's called *Actea -racemosa.* It's confusing.

Audience: Is this one quite angry as well?

Ian: It can be, but they tend to be more depressed than angry, for the most part. I've often confused it with *Sepia*. They often have this kind of heavy depression. They can also have anger, especially if they're in a lot of pain, you'll often see irritability and anger come out. It can be very painful. It seems to affect the nerves, inflame the nerves and so on. It's a good remedy.

Audience: Would you say that overall, they're more depressed than angry?

Ian: Generally, yes, it's stronger. They describe it like a black cloud. That's a typical *Cimicifuga* depression. Another one, I'm just thinking back, that I've used in sacroiliac problems is, I remember someone who was in a lot of pain, and it was *Colocynth*, again. There was the need to bend over, and that was the thing that relieved the pain. As long as he bent double, or half-double, he got relief. And when he straightened out, it was agony. And there was a lot of anger. So remember *Colocynth*. If someone's in a *Colocynth* state, these are the ones that you don't want to ask any questions really. It's not a good idea. Don't spend too long, and don't ask too many questions. It's like this person is angry, and they're worse if you question them, both *Colocynth* and *Nux-vomica*. They're like, "Just give me an Advil, will you?" It's like they haven't got the patience and they haven't got the threshold that they can think in terms of answering your questions. *Chamomilla* and *Coffea* can present a similar picture.

I'll just quickly mention, while we're on the back and so on, if someone has a problem since overlifting, that's probably the commonest aetiology for back strains and back problems, never well since overlifting. If that's the aetiology, you have to make sure that your remedy covers that. So there's a rubric in Murphy's *Repertory*, *"Ailments after overlifting,"* you'll see common remedies, *Arnica*, *Bryonia*, *Calc.-carb.*, which is often the underlying constitution, for someone who has a tendency to put their back out from overlifting, a tendency to strain them-selves. Also *Hypericum*, *Lycopodium*, and the strongest one, *Rhus.-tox.*, underline that, and then *Ruta*. (See page 125, *Back, Injuries, ailments after, lifting from*). It should be in that group. It has back trouble from overlifting. Those of you who are bodyworkers, you need to stock up on that little box of remedies. Learn the differentiations, and you should be able to prescribe them on the spot, pretty much.

Audience: If you're giving a remedy for that where there's not a real strong constitutional indication, would you give one dose, a single dose of 200 or something?

Ian: I would give at least a 200. When those backs go, they're in a lot of pain, usually. I can remember this from my own experience.

Audience: What about if it's a situation where the back goes out repeatedly, but you're not directly treating them for the pain, but for the tendency?

Ian: So what you look for then is a remedy that has a tendency to strains or overlifting injuries, and so on, which is a bigger group, which includes *Calc.-carb.* It includes *Rhus-tox*. It's also *Graphites* and other remedies. I used to work at a homeopathic college once, selling the books to the students. They used to have a little bookshop. I used to have to get up early on a Saturday morning and load this van with all these boxes of books that weighed a ton, and it was freezing cold, so I'm really tense and cold and huddled and my muscles are tight, and I bent down and I just felt my back go, and it was the first time that I had ever that happen, and it completely seized up, and I couldn't move. I couldn't straighten or anything, and of course I had just been studying *Rhus-tox.*, so I knew what remedy I needed. I overlifted and I was completely stiff and immobile, and I had a friend, I was sharing a flat at the time, and of course he's still in bed, it's like seven in the morning, I said, "Paul, throw me my kit - I need some remedies." Eventually, he wakes up. "What do you want?" *"Rhus-tox."* And he throws it to me out of the window, and I couldn't move to catch it. The whole thing was like a comedy show. I looked in the kit and I had *Rhus-tox.* 200. This was within five minutes of doing it, I took the remedy. It's still on my tongue, and I just felt this warmth go right down my back. The whole thing was just relaxed and eased. It was just amazing, the benefit of having the remedy on the spot. If I had waited three hours or so, it would probably have taken a day or two to heal, even with remedies. When you catch things on the spot like that, it hadn't fully crystallised in the body yet, so the remedy just blew it away, one dose, it was just amazing. I carried on lifting.

A while later, I had a similar thing happen. This is relatively recently, and this time, I was lifting something that didn't weigh anything. So that time, it was heavy boxes, right, and it was genuinely overlifting. More recently, I was lifting something that had some papers in it, and I put it down, and about five minutes later, my back went. So it wasn't while I was lifting and I didn't even lift anything heavy, but I kind of made an association. You know, I thought, "It must have been when I lifted that box," and it went into spasm. Now on this occasion, I took *Rhus-tox.* and it didn't do anything. Now the difference was, what I needed that second time was *Ignatia*. I was actually in an *Ignatia* state. I was upset about something which I hadn't really dealt with, so I was carrying that around, and just a tiny little thing was enough to bring out the picture.

I was teaching at college that weekend, and Beth, one of the teachers, she just looked at me, and she said, "Well, have you taken *Ignatia*?" "No - why, do you think I should?" She said, "Yes." And she looked in her kit, and she had *Ignatia* 30. As soon as I took that, I got immediate relief. So you can't get fixed in homeopathy, can you? What works one time won't work another. It seemed like the same scenario, but it wasn't, when I thought about it. One was genuine overlifting. The other, the predisposition was there from an emotional cause, and then just a little trigger was enough to set it off.

Audience: Have you ever found people for whom *Rhus-tox.* was a good constitutional?

Ian: Yes, I have, but I think it depends what you mean by constitutional. I've seen people where it's really helped them generally on every level, but in those cases, I think that, for the most part, they simply got stuck in a *Rhus-tox.* state. Something happened at some point in their life, and they acquired that state, as it were. And invariably, there'll be a constitutional remedy underneath that. Usually a *Calc.*, most typically. So they have a *Calc.* constitution and they overstrained, overlifted, got wet, got the flu, something happened, and they never fully recovered. And now they've needed *Rhus-tox.* ever since, on many levels. So I don't think they were truly a *Rhus-tox.* constitution, but it was their chronic remedy at the time. And I've seen the same with *Arnica* and *Hypericum*. I've seen *Arnica* work twenty years after an accident, and the person took it, and within minutes they felt the effect of it, and it was based on a twenty years ago aetiology. It's just amazing. The body can store things for so long, it's incredible.

Audience: I was noticing in the mentals of *Rhus*, the stiffness carries over into the mind and the emotions.

Ian: Right. That's what they say. And there's a side to *Rhus-tox.* that also has depression and suicidal tendencies and stuff.

Audience: The *Anacardium* side? It's related.

Ian: Right, botanically. And *Anacardium* is a big antidote to *Rhus* poisoning, isn't it? They're related in that respect. But I haven't seen *Rhus-tox.* on the mentals. I just haven't seen it. I'm not saying they don't exist, but I can't confirm it.

Let's just finish up here, before everybody falls asleep.

Audience: Earlier today, you were talking about muscles and tendons and ligaments, but now we're looking more locally like sacroiliac joint and things like that. What about an affinity to the shoulder?

Ian: There are some. I'll just mention a few, give you some tips, and then we'll have a quick look at some arthritic remedies.

One thing I learned with shoulders is that shoulder problems are often not shoulder problems. They're often coming from somewhere else, and one of the commonest places they're coming from is the gall bladder, which I've seen over and over and over. Not only the right shoulder, but most commonly the right. Anything that starts off in or is referred around the right shoulder blade, usually you've got a gall bladder problem. Frequently those things will travel up the right shoulder and into the neck. I've seen people having body work and stuff for months, and it's not working, and what they needed was a gall bladder remedy. *Chelidonium* usually, will cure that. So problems which originated in the right shoulder blade, particularly, *Chelidonium* will nearly always work.

Audience: In tincture?

Ian: I use it in potency in these cases, where there's a lot of pain and stuff. A few other tips on this.The right shoulder generally, the remedy with the strongest affinity is *Sanguinaria*. *Sanguinaria*, or Bloodroot, has the strongest affinity that I know of to the right shoulder. So if all the problems are referred there, and it often goes together with the right-sided headaches that *Sanguinaria* is famous for. So if you see that combination, especially. Right shoulder pains and right-sided headaches, that would be a good one to think of.

With the left shoulder, the strongest one that I've found is *Sulphur*. Pains and problems with the left shoulder, *Sulphur* has the strongest affinity. The other one on the right side that I should mention again is *Causticum*. Especially the right shoulder, right side of the neck, the whole right side of the body, *Causticum* is very strong there too.

Audience: Would this cover bursitis also?

Ian: Yes. And also, if it's bursitis, you'd have to include *Rhus-tox.* and *Ruta* in that group. More commonly with bursitis, there'll be an aetiology of lifting, using, exerting, straining, something like that. So if you get an aetiology, I would find a remedy that has the aetiology first, and the affinity second. So if you know it's from a strain or injury, make sure your remedy covers that first.

Audience: What if it's an allergic thing - this person I'm thinking of, whenever she eats something or other, she gets a horrible bursitis flare-up that takes a couple of weeks of really stringent management.

Ian: Does it swell up visibly?

Audience: I haven't seen it, but the way she talks about it, my impression is that there's swelling and mainly a lot of pain she talks about.

Ian: I'd think of *Apis*. It has an affinity with the joint capsules plus the tendency to swell plus the allergic reaction plus the worse for heat. A sticking pain would be nice. You could ask her a leading question. A couple of remedies for allergic response - *Apis* would be my number one. A second one is *Gentiana-lutea*, which you might not know so well. That's more for severe allergic reaction, bordering on anaphylaxis. *Apis* is more the urticaria or the localised oedema and swelling. Either they get hives, or they get a swelling up somewhere. And if nothing works, you've tried everything and it didn't work, and they know what food it is, then I would give them that food back, potentized. If it was just one thing, and it wasn't a whole range of things, and you've tried constitutional treatment, and you've tried *Apis*, and they're well in every other respect, but they still can't eat that one thing, then I'd give them that food, potentized. That's when I use isopathic prescriptions the most. It's like tidying up the loose ends. You treat constitutional, you've done the obvious, it still hasn't worked - go direct, use the local remedy.

Audience: So there's still, in this situation, there's not anything going on, you wouldn't see anything wrong with that, would you, to just to symptomatically do it?

Ian: I'd prefer to do it later rather than sooner. It tends to be more permanent if you do it to consolidate the cure, rather than in the beginning. That's been my experience. It's a bit like using pollen for hay fever. You know, you get potentized *Mixed pollen*, the person will have to keep taking it to get the relief. Whereas, if they have constitutional and miasmatic treatment, and then they have a dose of mixed pollen when they need it, it'll blow it away for the season. It's the difference between doing it first or doing it to tidy up the dregs. I try to encourage people to do it the other way around, but if they really won't have it, then I'll given them that. It's the patient's decision. I would try to educate the person to the point where they'll see the benefit of general treatment. If they don't want it, who am I to say?

Audience: Or if it it's not working?

Ian: Yes, if it's not working, you could try to go direct. And Kent did this as well, he advocated this. He talks about cases, where a person's allergic to strawberries, or something, and he tried remedies that didn't work, then he'd give them potentized strawberry and it cured the case. So you've got it on the highest authority, if you need it!

Just a couple of remedies for cellulitis. That's a nasty disease. A person gets an infection in the cellular tissues and they usually end up on heavy antibiotics and stuff. I saw a couple of really nasty cases of that when I was away in Egypt, working in Cairo, and I saw a woman who came in and her leg was out to here, and it was diagnosed as cellulitis, and she was on heavy antibiotics, and the remedy was *Lachesis*, in her case. It was all purplish and bluish, worse for heat, and she had a dose of *Lachesis* 200, and got completely cured. A couple of days, it was all gone. It was amazing. The other top remedies I've seen in cellulitis are *Apis* and *Rhus-tox..* They're the two main ones that have an affinity with the intercellular tissues. I would add *Lachesis* to that group, and also *Mercurius*.

Now just a couple of tips on treating arthritis generally. One thing I would recommend is that I get better results with arthritis if I find a general remedy which also covers the arthritis. You know, it's a systemic disease, even if it's affecting only the knees, wrists, or whatever. I prefer not to just find a 'wrists' remedy, if it's diagnosed as arthritis. It's a degenerative condition. What I look for is a constitutional which has an affinity with the fingers or the wrists or the knees, whatever is affected. Failing that, then I'll go for a local remedy. But that's my preference.

Probably, if there's one remedy I've used successfully more often than any other remedy in rheumatoid arthritis, it would be *Natrum-mur*. So that would be my number one remedy for rheumatoid arthritis. In Cumbria, in the Lake District, where I live, it's a damp climate. There's a lot of arthritic, rheumatic people, so it's something that was worth specialising in, getting reasonably good at treating, and I found that a huge percentage of arthritic patients would benefit from *Nat.-mur*. It wouldn't cure them all, but they would invariably get relief from it, and many, it would cure, if I kept with it for long enough. It has all the symptoms that are common to arthritis: pain, stiffness, swelling in the joints, and often the temperament that goes together with it, the tendency to be reserved, withdrawn, and with suppressed grief, resentment, or something of that kind. Often there's a holding onto something with arthritis, which is manifesting in the joints.

Audience: What was your potency approach?

Ian: Low and often, so a 6C, three times a day, and then keeping them on it for months, if necessary. It's a slow moving disease, usually, so the treatment should be slow and progressive. I'd rather do it that way than whack them with a high potency. It's much less dramatic, and much more effective in the long term. If you see arthritis in the fingers, a couple of main remedies there. One is *Caulophylum*, especially if you see it since menopause, pregnancy, or other hormonal change. Arthritis affecting the hands and fingers in a woman, where there's a hormonal link - *Caulophylum*. If there isn't a hormonal link and it's the fingers, look at *Staphysagria*. Big, big remedy in arthritis, *Staphysagria*, especially when they get nodosities, the fingers start getting all deformed and disfigured.

Audience: Does it have any contractures, too?

Ian: I haven't seen it cure that.

Audience: It's just nodules?

Ian: Yes, but sometimes people will need it. You know, it's got to the point where they've got contractures. They may still benefit from *Staph.*, but I haven't seen it actually help to straighten contractures. But what you should remember is that the complementary of *Staph.* is *Causticum.* It will often go into *Causticum.* Also, get these people using castor oil if it's the hands and the fingers, rubbed in, every morning, every night. And they like it, I find that people like something to do, especially the older people. They really benefit. Every morning, every night, they do their castor oil, and you get them doing their chi kung finger rolls, which are very helpful, and amazingly effective. Even if you don't get the right remedies, they'll come back better, if they're doing this every morning, every night they'll feel improvement, and it buys you time to figure out your remedies.

Arthritis in the hips - *Nat.-mur.*, again, *Kali-carb.*, we mentioned already. The *Calciums*, especially *Calc.-carb.*, and *Calc.-fluor.*, have a strong affinity with the hips.

Audience: *Aurum* can have a hip arthritis, can't it?

Ian: Yes. *Aurum* you'll see more often in the osteoarthritis than the rheumatoid arthritis, because of the bone affinity.

Audience: It's a more common arthritis, the osteo.....

Ian: I think it depends on where you live, to be honest. There's probably more of the rheumatic type, where I used to live. Here you might look more at the *Calcium* salts and the *Phosphorus* salts and the *Aurums*, the different *Aurums*, such as *Aurum-mur.*, *Aurum-met.* etc.

Audience: How about *Sulphur?*

Ian: *Sulphur*, yes. *Sulphur* is a big remedy in arthritis, and its easily overlooked. I've often missed it. A few other ones just to think about. This is when it is affecting the knees in particular, *Berberis-vulgaris.* This is a kidney support remedy, and can be very, very helpful for osteoarthritis. If you improve the elimination by the kidneys, very often the osteoarthritis will be alleviated. I've seen that especially true where it's either in the back, arthritis in the spine, and or the knees, *Berberis-vulgaris.* It'll often stimulate the kidney function, so you should tell the patient that, "Don't be surprised if you start urinating frequently," and it's a good sign. The urine will often go cloudy for a while, and the joints will improve.

Audience: Is that in tincture?

Ian: Yes. I use it in tincture or just very low potency, either way. And also, don't forget *Medorrhinum.* Many cases of arthritis won't really make a big improvement until they get *Medorrhinum.* That's more the sycotic cases, so you'll see, typical things will be the damp affects them, either aggravation or amelioration from damp. There will be a relationship to damp, one way or another. If they tell you they're better by the sea, it's even better. That's a great indication for *Medorrhinum*. Also, people that tell you that it came on since they moved location. You know, they've moved from the coast, or they moved inland, or to the lakes, or something. I've seen lots of people who retired to the Lakes, because it's a place that people want to retire to. They go there for their holidays, and then when they quit their job, they move there. And they're in good health and they have all these visions of walking up the mountains and so on, and within six months of getting there, their joints start to seize up. This is *Medorrhinum*. It's the sycotic miasm being woken up, just by the climatic change. It has nothing to do with emotional trauma or anything. It's an environmental aetiology. So I use *Medorrhinum* very, very frequently in arthritis, in the elderly people as well as the not so elderly.

Audience: In both types, the rheumatoid and the osteoarthritis?

Ian: Yes. Mostly in the rheumatoid, but both types can need it.

Don't forget *Rhus-tox.*, especially if you get a lot of stiffness as the strongest symptom, worse damp, better for heat.

Audience: What about *Arsenicum?*

Ian: Yes. Burning pains, restlessness with the pains. Most of the polychrests you'll see can be needed. If you look at arthritis in the repertory, it's a big rubric, with every big remedy. *Pulsatilla*, you'll see, better movement, worse heat. A little one I've seen quite often, *Rhododendron*, that's an interesting one. That's more the rheumatic type. These are the people who can predict the weather changes. They feel when it's going to rain. They can feel it in their joints. This is *Rhododendron*. These are a few clues. There are many, many more remedies, but you can do a lot with arthritis. What I usually look for is a general remedy which has an affinity with the weakest point in the person, whether it's the hips, or whatever. If it's generalised and wandering around, then you want a wandering around remedy. It could be *Tuberculinum, Pulsatilla, Kalmia-latifolia*, something like that. So the nature of it can determine the remedy. It's a big topic. If it's changing sides, think of *Lac-caninum*. I've seen *Lac-caninum* help rheumatism. One time, it would be worse on the right, next time, worse on the left, and you don't quite know what to do, give them *Lac-caninum*. Another one I've seen with severe hip pains is *Stramonium*. That's one that surprised me, but it worked really well. If they have a pain like someone's sticking a knife in the hip, it sounds pretty *Stramonium*-like doesn't it?

Audience: Is that the left hip?

Ian: Is it the left? I don't remember, but it's real specific if someone has a sharp, stabbing pain in the hip. *Datura-stramonium.* It's pretty heavy stuff.

Well, we could go on, but there's always more, so I think we'll call it a day. Thanks for coming along. I hope you got something you can take away and use, and I'm sure that the rest will be filed away for future reference.

Therapeutic Index

About the Author

Ian Watson is co-founder of The Lakeland College and author of *A Guide to the Methodologies of Homeopathy* and *The Tao of Homeopathy.* He lives in Devon with his wife and daughter, and is known internationally as a lecturer and workshop leader in the fields of homeopathy and self-development.

For details of Ian's other writings, recorded seminars and forthcoming events, visit:
www.ianwatsonseminars.com

Lightning Source UK Ltd.
Milton Keynes UK
UKOW051111140113

204838UK00001B/257/A